Recent Results in Cancer Research   112

Founding Editor
P. Rentchnick, Geneva

Managing Editors
Ch. Herfarth, Heidelberg · H.-J. Senn, St. Gallen

Associate Editors
M. Baum, London · V. Diehl, Köln
C. von Essen, Villigen · E. Grundmann, Münster
W. Hitzig, Zürich · M. F. Rajewsky, Essen

Recent Results in Cancer Research

Volume 102: Epidemiology of Malignant Melanoma
Edited by R. P. Gallagher
1986. 15 figures, 70 tables. IX, 169. ISBN 3-540-16020-5

Volume 103: Preoperative (Neoadjuvant) Chemotherapy
Edited by J. Ragaz, P. R. Band, J. H. Goldie
1986. 58 figures, 49 tables. IX, 162. ISBN 3-540-16129-5

Volume 104: Hyperthermia and the Therapy of Malignant Tumors
Edited by C. Streffer
1987. 52 figures, 63 tables. IX, 207. ISBN 3-540-17250-5

Volume 105: Breast Cancer
Edited by S. Brünner and B. Langfeldt
1987. 59 figures, 43 tables. IX, 132. ISBN 3-540-17301-3

Volume 106: Minimal Neoplasia
Edited by E. Grundmann and L. Beck
1988. 128 figures, 61 tables. IX, 194. ISBN 3-540-18455-4

Volume 107: Application of Hyperthermia
in the Treatment of Cancer
Edited by R. D. Issels and W. Wilmanns
1988. 118 figures, 56 tables. XII, 277. ISBN 3-540-18486-4

Volume 108: Supportive Care in Cancer Patients
Edited by H.-J. Senn, A. Glaus, L. Schmid
1988. 62 figures, 97 tables. ISBN 3-540-17150-9

Volume 109: Preclinical Hyperthermia
Edited by W. Hinkelbein, G. Bruggmoser, R. Engelhardt
1988. 182 figures, 40 tables. ISBN 3-540-18487-2

Volume 110: Combined Modality Therapy of Gastrointestinal
Tract Cancer
Edited by P. Schlag, P. Hohenberger, U. Metzger
1988. 105 figures, 122 tables. ISBN 3-540-18610-7

Volume 111: Cancer Clinical Trials: A Critical Appraisal
Edited by H. Scheurlen, R. Kay, M. Baum
1988. 37 figures, 53 tables. XI, 272. ISBN 3-540-19098-8

L. Schmid H.-J. Senn (Eds.)

AIDS-Related Neoplasias

With 23 Figures and 35 Tables

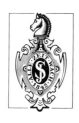

Springer-Verlag
Berlin Heidelberg New York
London Paris Tokyo

Dr. Luzius Schmid
Prof. Dr. Hans-Jörg Senn

Medizinische Klinik C, Kantonsspital St. Gallen
9007 St. Gallen, Switzerland

ISBN 3-540-19227-1 Springer-Verlag Berlin Heidelberg New York
ISBN 0-387-19227-1 Springer-Verlag New York Berlin Heidelberg

Library of Congress Cataloging-in-Publication Data.
AIDS-related neoplasias/L. Schmid, H.-J. Senn (eds.). p. cm. – (Recent results in
cancer research; 112) Includes bibliographies and index.
ISBN 0-387-19227-1 (U.S.)
1. AIDS (Disease)-Congresses. 2. Cancer-Etiology-Congresses. 3. Kaposi's sarcoma-Con-
gresses. 4. Lymphomas-Congresses.
I. Schmid, L. II. Senn, Hansjörg. III. Series.
[DNLM: 1. Acquired Immunodeficiency Syndrome-complications. 2. Neoplasms-com-
plications. W1 RE106P v.112/ WD 308 A28846]
RC261.R35 vol. 112 [RC607.A26] 616.99'4 s-dc 19 [616.99'4071] DNLM/DLC
88-16084

© Springer-Verlag Berlin Heidelberg 1988
Printed in Germany

The use of registered names, trademarks, etc. in this publication does not imply, even in the
absence of a specific statement, that such names are exempt from the relevant protective
laws and regulations and therefore free for general use.

Product Liability: The publisher can give no guarantee for information about drug dosage
and application thereof contained in the book. In every individual case the respective user
must check its accuracy by consulting other pharmaceutical literature.

Typesetting, printing, and binding: Appl, Wemding
2125/3140-543210

Preface

The acquired immunodeficiency syndrome (AIDS) and the AIDS-related complex (ARC) are caused by the human immunodeficiency virus (HIV-I), previously known as human T-cell lymphotropic virus type III (HTLV-III) or lymphadenopathy-associated virus (LAV). It seems that additional retroviruses (HIV-II and perhaps others) are able to cause variants of AIDS or ARC.[1-3]

Patients infected with the virus may (but do not necessarily) develop a wide range of clinical symptoms that are not directly related to the virus itself, but are secondary to the devastating effects of the viral infection on the human immune system. The virus thus renders the patient susceptible to a variety of opportunistic infections with other viruses (such as cytomegalovirus), bacteria, fungi, and protozoa, as well as to the development of simultaneous or subsequent malignant tumors.

The new topic of AIDS and cancer is a challenging and frightening aspect of present-day medicine and health politics. With the growing prevalence of the human immunodeficiency virus(es) and clinical correlates ranging from persistent generalized lymphadenopathy (PGL) to full-blown AIDS in our population, we will also encounter a steadily rising number of patients with *both* AIDS and neoplasias, such as Kaposi's sarcoma, Hodgkin's and non-Hodgkin's lymphomas, anal cancer, and a variety of additional malignant tumors.[4, 5]

---

[1] Gallo RC, Salahuddin SZ, Popvic M et al. (1984) Frequent detection and isolation of cytopathic retroviruses (HTLV-III) from patients with AIDS and at risk for AIDS. Science 224: 500–503.

[2] Montagnier L, Gruest J, Charamet S et al. (1984) Adaption of lymphadenopathy associated virus to replication in EBV transformed B lymphoblastic cell lines. Science 251: 1447–1449.

[3] Coffin J, Hasse A, Levy J et al. (1986) What to call the AIDS virus. Nature 321: 10.

[4] Kaplan MH, Susin M, Pahwa SG et al. (1987) Neoplastic complications of HTLV-III infection. Am J Med 82: 389–396.

[5] Groopman JE (1987) Neoplasms in the acquired immune deficiency syndrome: the multidisciplinary approach to treatment. Semin Oncol 14 [Suppl 3] 1–6.

The rapid rise in the number of patients with these malignancies and HIV seropositivity in United States cancer centers during the past 2–3 years is predictive of what will take place in European cities and tumor centers within the next 3–5 years. Are we, as "health professionals" (doctors, nurses, and social workers), and our health care politicians, *prepared* to meet this growing challenge within the framework of our present medical and nursing structures? If not, how must we then proceed in the very near future, given the significant differences in epidemiologic, political, and socioeconomic conditions in various countries and cities throughout Europe?

The purpose of this workshop was specifically to unite oncologists and hematologists (and related personnel such as nurses and social workers) with clinical experience in dealing with HIV-infected patients and neoplastic disease. The meeting represented the first public action of the recently formed working party for AIDS-associated tumors of the Swiss Group for Clinical Cancer Research (SAKK). Together with oncologists from surrounding countries – France, Germany, and Italy – we have felt the need to discuss strategies of how to deal with the growing problem of AIDS and cancer.

Possible solutions cannot be confined to the medical level, but must also involve nursing, psychosocial, and economic aspects. Who in the framework of modern medicine is better prepared to meet the challenge of AIDS and cancer than medical oncologists and hematooncologists with their affiliated nurses, who – by virtue of their training and experience with immunocompromised hosts and with palliative care – have a long-standing record of dealing with similar patient problems in the past?

Above all, we would like to sensitize health officials and hospital boards to the growing problem of AIDS and cancer. This book should clarify some of the controversy about the magnitude of the problem, as well as about the possibilities of presently available treatments of malignant disease in HIV-seropositive patients, and will, we hope, encourage the setting up of international prospective clinical trials in the very near future.

St. Gallen, June 1988   H.-J. Senn

Contents

B. Somaini, J. Bleuer, and H. Vorkauf
AIDS in Central Europe 1

J. Schüpbach
The Etiology of AIDS and Its Relevance for AIDS-Related
Neoplasias 6

*E. M. Hersh, E. A. Petersen, D. E. Yocum, S. R. Gorman,
M. J. Darragh, C. R. Gschwind, G. W. Brewton, and J. A. Reuben*
Immunological Characteristics and Potential Approaches
to Immunotherapy of HIV Infection 17

A. E. Friedman-Kien
AIDS-Related Kaposi's Sarcoma 27

S. Monfardini
Malignant Lymphomas in Patients with or at Risk for AIDS
in Italy 37

*J.-M. Andrieu, M. Toledano, M. Raphael, J.-M. Tourani,
and B. Desablens*
HIV-Related Hematological Neoplasias in France 46

E. M. Hersh and T. P. Miller
Malignant Lymphomas in Patients with Human
Immunodeficiency Virus Infection 54

D. Huhn and M. Serke
Malignant Lymphomas and HIV Infection 63

L. Schmid
AIDS-Related Neoplasias in Switzerland 69

B. R. Saltzman and A. E. Friedman-Kien
Inactivation of HIV and Safety Precautions for the Workplace 75

H. Christ
Psychosocial Issues for Patients with AIDS-Related Cancers . 84

L. Schmid
Summary and Future Prospects 93

Subject Index 94

List of Contributors*

Andrieu, J.-M. *46*[1]
Bleuer, J. *1*
Brewton, G.W. *17*
Christ, H. *84*
Darragh, M.J. *17*
Desablens, B. *46*
Friedman-Kien, A.E. *27, 75*
Gorman, S.R. *17*
Gschwind, C.R. *17*
Hersh, E.M. *17, 54*
Huhn, D. *63*
Miller, T.P. *54*
Monfardini, S. *37*

Petersen, E.A. *17*
Raphael, M. *46*
Reuben, J.A. *17*
Saltzman, B.R. *75*
Schmid, L. *69, 93*
Schüpbach, J. *6*
Serke, M. *63*
Somaini, B. *1*
Toledano, M. *46*
Tourani, J.-M. *46*
Vorkauf, H. *1*
Yocum, D.E. *17*

---

* The address of the principal author is given on the first page of each contribution.
[1] Page on which contribution begins.

AIDS in Central Europe

B. Somaini, J. Bleuer, and H. Vorkauf

Federal Office of Public Health, 3001 Bern, Switzerland

The clinical pattern of AIDS was first described in 1981. Routine proof of an HIV infection did not become possible before mid-1985, although the virus was first described in 1983 [6]. As a consequence, all epidemiological knowledge about AIDS and the HIV infection is merely a few years old. Nevertheless, it is astounding how much has been learned about the infection in such a short time. However, it has only recently been possible to improve documentation about the distribution of HIV in various parts of the world. A great deal still remains unclear. Any survey is based on the current state of observation, and this may already be outdated after a few months; by the time AIDS statistics are published, they are already outdated. Even so, the recorded number of existing AIDS cases provides important information and often constitutes a basis for further activities.

An AIDS diagnosis is made with the help of clearly defined clinical criteria. These criteria changed only insignificantly between 1982 and 1987, and it is therefore possible to produce a trend analysis on the basis of reported cases.

Increase in Cases of AIDS

In Europe it was decided as early as 1983 to report all cases of AIDS centrally. This wise decision now makes possible the evaluation of trends over the past 4 years (Fig. 1). By end of June 1983, 153 cases of AIDS had been reported in Europe. Today, 4 years later, the figure stands at 6500 AIDS cases [9].

On the basis of these data it is evident that:

- Most of these cases belong to the age group of 20- to 40-year-olds, and that the ratio of men to women is about 10:1.
- The number of cases has been steadily rising over the past 4 years.
- A continuous increase at a similar rate is to be feared in the coming years.

As regards the factor of time, the United States has a "head start" of 2–3 years over Europe. But a comparison of European with American figures demonstrates a striking similarity, the only difference consisting in the time lag of the former. For Europe, estimates predict that over 25 000 cases of AIDS will have been registered by the end of 1988 [1].

Recent Results in Cancer Research, Vol. 112
© Springer-Verlag Berlin · Heidelberg 1988

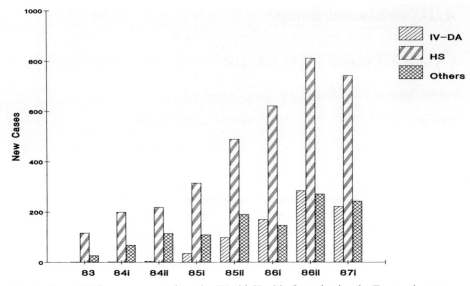

Fig. 1. New AIDS cases reported to the World Health Organization in Europe by transmission group and by half-year of reporting, as of March 1987. *IV-DA*, intravenous drug addicts; *HS*, homosexual and bisexual men; *others*, haemophiliacs, transfusion-associated cases, heterosexual transmission, etc.

Trends Among Certain Population Groups

Homosexuals. Since 1981 homosexuals have been most affected by the disease. In Europe, the proportion of homosexuals suffering from AIDS has hardly changed, and homosexuals currently account for some 65% of all AIDS patients. The total number of cases has risen from somewhat over 100 in 1983 to over 4000 in 1987 [9].

Intravenous Drug Addicts. In Europe, the first AIDS diagnoses among intravenous drug users were not made until 1984. The rise in the number of cases among this population group is alarming (Fig. 1). The mathematical model of the World Health Organization (WHO) centre in Paris [1] predicts some 15000 AIDS patients among intravenous drug users by the end of 1988. These estimates contain a wide margin of uncertainty; however, experience gained in the first 6 months of 1987 confirms the extrapolation to date. On the basis of these observations, we fear that this forecast will become reality. It should be noted that up to now reports on drug-addicted AIDS patients come predominantly from southern Europe.

Heterosexual Population. To date, only some 4% of all reported cases have occurred through heterosexual transmission. It is not easy, however, to define the heterosexual risk precisely. The number of heterosexuals with AIDS is slowly but steadily rising. It is important to point out that in all persons except those with exclusively homosexual relationships heterosexual contacts do occur, for instance, in

Table 1. AIDS cases and heterosexual transmission in Switzerland (to March 1987)

	Number of cases	Age	Sexual contacts with
Men	4	28, 31, 41, 61	Women from Africa or Haiti
	1	61	Prostitutes
	1	31	Female drug addict
Women	2	21, 49	Men from Africa or Haiti
	1	26	Frequently changing male partners (prostitution)
	1	49	Man from America with multiple prostitute contacts
	1	24	Bisexual man
	1	35	Male AIDS patient

bisexual men and intravenous drug users. Current European data do not well document heterosexual transmission. But as regards Switzerland, out of a total of 221 cases reported by end of March 1987 only 5% belong to this category [5], excluding persons from Africa and the Caribbean (Table 1). The distribution between the sexes in heterosexual cases is virtually 1:1.

Spectrum of Symptoms

Regarding the spectrum of symptoms, 4 years of experience in Europe allows certain generalisations. From the outset the disease has been roughly classified as opportunistic infection, Kaposi's sarcoma, Kaposi's sarcoma with opportunistic infection, and other clinical patterns. If the reports are grouped according to symptom groups, it becomes clear that the respective proportions have remained relatively steady. However, it cannot be overlooked that in the group "others" further clinical manifestations, including tumours, are appearing with increasing frequency [9].

Comparing the spectrum among drug users with that among others (mostly homosexuals), it is striking, that Kaposi's sarcoma is seldom found among drug users (Fig. 2) and is encountered predominantly among homosexuals. Other tumours, however, are found in all groups.

The Current Problem and Prospects for the Future

It would be very mistaken to base planning and preventive measures on the current pattern of prevalence and incidence of AIDS cases. People who became ill in 1986, for instance, were infected already several years ago, and as a consequence they were potentially infectious for many years and may have infected other people over this period [4].

Small-scale studies estimate that some 7 years after infection one-third of those who are seropositive have developed AIDS, one-third show other HIV-associated

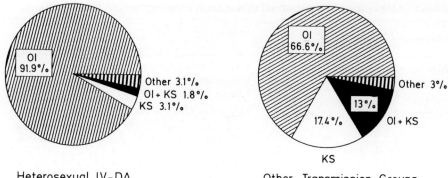

Fig. 2. Disease category in AIDS cases in intravenous drug addicts *(IV-DA)* and other transmission groups in Europe to March 1987 [9]. *KS,* Kaposi's sarcoma; *OI,* opportunistic infection

symptoms, and one-third are clear of symptoms [3]. To what extent these findings will be confirmed in the future, and how many more persons will progress to AIDS 10 or 20 years after infection are unknown [2]. But let us take this distribution hypothetically as final and take another look at the past. Today we know of some 6000 recorded AIDS cases in Europe. Assuming that this figure comprises only one-third of those infected 7 years ago, there would already have been 18000 seropositive persons in Europe in 1980, although AIDS was not even known at that time. Since then the virus has spread, at first without being known, and is still spreading. Today we estimate a few hundred thousand infected persons in Europe. In 7 years probably one-third of these will have developed AIDS, and a further one-third will have contracted other HIV-associated illnesses. This is in itself a major problem, but the fact that all these people are potentially infectious creates even a greater problem. The most important mode of transmission is sexual intercourse. To prevent this epidemic we must focus our intervention in this area.

As a result of the long incubation period there is an unknown number of already infected persons who do not yet show any symptoms. From the beginning of the epidemic the number of patients in the preliminary phase compared to the number of AIDS cases has been relatively high. However, only with the testing procedures which became available 2 years ago has it become possible to determine the number of virus carriers who do not show any symptoms and thus to make the alarming assessment of how far and how insidiously the virus has spread.

Today's figures on the prevalence of AIDS therefore reflect the infection level around 1980; the current infection rate will not be manifested in AIDS statistics for many years. It is always later than we think - it is often too late. The difficulty begins with the task of making it clear to the general public that an epidemic is in progress. Such motivational problems did not arise in the past, for example with the plague or cholera, because the extent of the catastrophe was always immediately recognizable for everyone. It is now clear that the extent of the epidemic is determined by the number of virus carriers, and that there is a risk of infection for all who exposes themselves to certain dangerous situations: risky sexual contacts and sharing syringes and other instruments when injecting drugs.

Because of their specifically high-risk behaviour those practising homosexuality and intravenous drug injection predominate among AIDS cases in Europe. However, this must not allow us to be misled: any unprotected sexual intercourse with an infected person entails a risk of infection. Anal intercourse probably constitutes a higher risk than vaginal intercourse [2]. In Europe and the United States the likelihood of encountering an infected heterosexual partner is significantly lower than that of encountering an infected homosexual partner. As a consequence the disease is still spreading less rapidly among the heterosexual population. But as more persons become infected, it will spread more rapidly, and it is at this point that we must concentrate all our efforts at prevention.

Sexual transmission can already be significantly controlled [7]. For all sexually active persons who do not live in a long-term, monogamous, two-person partnership with an uninfected partner, there are two possibilities:

1. Sexual abstinence. Thousands of years of experience, however, show that this life-style is not a long-term solution.
2. Sexual contacts only with condoms. The correct use of good-quality condoms provides very effective protection [8].

These simple recommendations must reach all persons exposed to potential risk, even though the risk of heterosexual transmission is currently rather low. Each infection we prevent today will prevent many infections in the future.

References

1. Downs A, Ancelle R, Jager H, Brunet J (1987) AIDS in Europe: current trends and short-term predictions estimated from surveillance data, January 1981–June 1986. AIDS 1: 53–57
2. Francis DP, Chin J (1987) The prevention of AIDS in United States; an objective strategy for medicine, public health, business and the community. JAMA 257: 1357–1366
3. Hessol N, Rutherford G, O'Malley P, Doll L, Darrow W, Jaffe H (1987) The natural history of HIV-infection in a cohort of homosexual and bisexual men: a 7-year prospective study. Presented at the 3rd international conference on AIDS, Washington D.C., June 1–5, p 1
4. Institute of Medicine, National Academy of Sciences (1986) Confronting AIDS: directions for public health, health care and research. National Academy Press, Washington D.C.
5. Janett A, Stutz T, Somaini B, Vorkauf H, Kaufmann M (1987) Heterosexual transmission of HIV in Switzerland. Presented at the 3rd international conference on AIDS, Washington D.C., June 1–5, p 19
6. Meyer K, Pauker S (1987) Screening for HIV: can we afford the false positive rate? New Engl J Med 317: 238–241
7. Somaini B, Stutz T, Janett A (1987) Information und Prävention. Soz Praventivmed 32: 15–17
8. Van de Perre P, Jacobs D, Sprecher S (1987) The latex condom, an efficient barrier against sexual transmission of AIDS-related viruses. AIDS 1: 49–52
9. WHO Collaborating Centre on AIDS (1987) AIDS surveillance in Europe, Report no 13. WHO, Paris

The Etiology of AIDS and Its Relevance for AIDS-Related Neoplasias

J. Schüpbach

Nationales Zentrum für Retroviren, Institut für Immunologie und Virologie, Universität Zürich, Gloriastraße 30, 8028 Zürich, Switzerland

Introduction

A high incidence of malignancy is seen in various congenital and acquired immunodeficiency diseases. Ataxia telangiectasia and Wiskott-Aldrich syndrome are associated with the development of cancer in 11.7% and 15.4% of patients, respectively. Most of these malignancies are B-cell immunoblastic, non-Hodgkin's lymphomas, and many have primary location in the central nervous system, as compared with only 2% in the general population. Recipients of renal transplants receiving immunosuppressive therapy have a 2%–13% incidence of malignancy, the average time between transplantation and cancer diagnosis being 16 months to 3 years [39].

The tumors seen in association with AIDS fit well into this pattern. Apparently, the state of severe immunodeficiency is sufficient for the genesis, by various etiologic factors, of malignant tumors. This paper will briefly review the viruses etiologically associated with AIDS, describe in more detail the mechanisms of immunopathogenesis, and, finally, give some consideration to the currently most frequently seen tumors, Kaposi's sarcoma (KS) and non-Hodgkin's lymphoma (NHL).

Classification of Human Immunodeficiency Viruses

Human immunodeficiency viruses (HIV), a family of related lentiviruses etiologically associated with the acquired immunodeficiency syndrome (AIDS), now include at least two and possibly three different types (Fig. 1). The "classical" isolates comprise those viruses originally isolated from patients with AIDS and related diseases and variably designated as LAV, HTLV-III, or ARV, which were identified as the etiologic agents of AIDS in 1984 [2, 7, 36, 41, 44, 26]. These viruses, now referred to as HIV-1, are responsible for the current AIDS epidemic in central Africa, Europe, the Americas, and other regions of the world. A novel type of HIV, HIV-2, was identified as LAV-2 in AIDS patients of West African origin [4] and as HTLV-IV in healthy prostitutes of this region [18]. Its progress in Europe and the United States appears to be slow, and at the moment HIV-2 is not of quantitative importance in these areas. A third type of AIDS-associated viruses, distantly related to HIV-2, was recently identified in Nigerian patients with disease similar to AIDS; this virus will likely be termed HIV-3 (R.C. Gallo, commu-

Recent Results in Cancer Research, Vol. 112
© Springer-Verlag Berlin·Heidelberg 1988

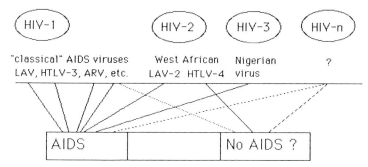

Fig. 1. Classification of human immunodeficiency viruses. The figure includes possible additional virus types *(HIV-n)* and the possible existence of virus isolates which may be devoid of a pathogenic effect

nication at the 3rd international conference on AIDS, Washington D.C., June 1–5, 1987).

It is still a matter of debate as to whether LAV-2 and HTLV-IV differ in their pathogenic potential. While LAV-2 is clearly associated with AIDS [3,5], HTLV-IV is claimed not to cause AIDS. This latter suggestion is based on the observation of a high prevalence of antibodies, in the absence of symptoms suggestive of immunodeficiency, in some West African populations, ranging from 1%–10% in the population at large to 15%–65% in prostitutes. This high frequency suggests that the virus may have been present in that region for a long period of time. If it had a pathogenic effect, disease should have become manifest. However, seropositive prostitutes observed now for 2 years have not developed lymphadenopathy or clinical symptoms of AIDS. In addition, the prevalence of antibodies reactive with HTLV-IV was not higher in patients with infectious diseases, suggesting that infection with this virus does not predispose to opportunistic infections (M. Essex, communication at the 3rd international conference on AIDS). However, the lack of overt disease may also be attributable to a long incubation period. The situation may be similar to that in Kenya, where infection among prostitutes was documented long before the first cases of AIDS appeared [24].

Genome and Proteins of HIV

A schematic representation of the genome and the proteins of HIV-1 is given in Fig. 2. As all retroviruses, HIV has two genes that code for structural proteins, *gag* for proteins of the core and *env* for proteins of the viral envelope. *Pol* codes for the enzyme reverse transcriptase. The final proteins, as well as the precursors from which they are derived, are shown in the light boxes of Fig. 2 surrounding the shaded genome box.

In addition to the three obligatory genes, HIV possesses a number of regulatory genes *(tat, art, 3'orf)*. The regulatory proteins govern the expression of both structural and regulatory genes and are responsible for the insiduous propagation of the virus that leads to a slowly progressive disease, characterized by alternating phases of active virus replication and latency.

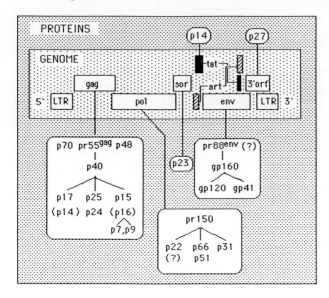

Fig. 2. Schematic representation of the genome and the proteins of HIV-1. (From [52])

Furthermore, the genome contains additional genes (e.g., the *R* gene located in the region between *pol* and *env* and other possibly coding open-reading frames. Their function is not known, and they are therefore not shown in Fig. 2. The genomes of all retroviruses are flanked by regulatory sequences, the long terminal repeats (LTR). They contain signals for initiation and enhancement of transmission. In HIV the action of the LTR is greatly enhanced by the binding of the *tat* protein.

All structural as well as regulatory gene products are immunogenic and lead to the formation of antibodies in almost all infected persons. This feature is not only important for the diagnosis of HIV infection but may also play a role in the pathogenesis of the disease (see below).

Pathogenesis of AIDS

The in vitro cytopathogenic effect of HIV is well documented. Certain concepts and preliminary evidence suggest that host factors may also be important in the pathogenesis of AIDS.

The most important effector systems of the immune defense – production of antibodies, cytotoxic T-lymphocytes (CTL) and natural killer cells, monocytes/macrophages – require the assistance of helper T cells which exhibit the surface marker CD4 (also called T4). This assistance consists of lymphokines produced and secreted by T4 cells, most important of which are interleukin 2 (IL-2) and γ-interferon (IFN). T4 cells produce and secrete these lymphokines only when they themselves are activated. Under natural circumstances activation results from presentation of foreign antigens (from viruses, bacteria, fungi). These antigens are ingested and modified (processed) by monocytes/macrophages and other antigen-presenting cells (APC) and then expressed at their surface in conjunction with MHC-

II (a class II molecule of the major histocompatibility complex). The antigen/ MHC-II complex is recognized by the antigen receptor of the T4 cell. For activation a second signal is required, in the form of interleukin 1 (IL-1) secreted by the APC. In addition, the close contact required for these recognition processes is probably dependent on interaction of the CD4 molecule and the nonpolymorphic part of MHC-II. These processes are schematically presented in Fig. 3.

The central immune defect of AIDS patients consists of the inability of T4 cells to recognize soluble antigen presented to them [25]. This inability results in the failure of all T helper cell dependent effector systems. There are several different pathways by which HIV infection interferes, or might interfere, with the processes of antigen recognition and T4 cell activation.

Viral Effects on HIV-Infected Cells. HIV may infect not only T4 cells but also cells of the monocyte/macrophage lineage and other APC. Possibly, these cells are even the first target of HIV in the course of infection [8, 19, 22, 27, 33]. The close contact required for antigen presentation is likely to facilitate cell-to-cell transmission of HIV.

HIV infection of these cells is mediated by the CD4 molecule which acts as a virus receptor [6, 20]. Productive infection of CD4-positive cells leads to cell death. The cytopathic effect appears to be dependent on both the viral gp120 envelope protein and the density of cellular CD4. Possibly, virus budding from the surface

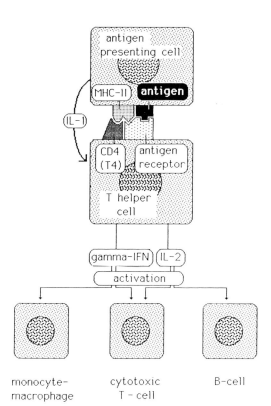

Fig. 3. Schematic representation of the processes of antigen recognition by T4-cells. (From [52])

monocyte-macrophage   cytotoxic T - cell   B-cell

of infected cells interacts with CD4 molecules on the same cells and thus leads to autofusion (Haseltine, communication at the 3rd international conference on AIDS). As monocytes have a lower density of surface CD4, they may be more resistant to HIV than T4 cells and may survive longer after infection. As an additional mechanism, cell fusion between infected cells expressing gp120 and uninfected CD4-positive cells has been postulated [28, 46]. This leads to the generation of syncytia resulting in premature cell death. Both mechanisms lead to the death of the two cells principally involved in antigen recognition. In addition, HIV infection of T4 cells appears to down-regulate the expression of IL-2 in T4 cells (C. Lane, F. Wong-Staal, communications at the 3rd international conference on AIDS).

Antiviral Immune Responses Against HIV-Infected or -Coated Cells. Cells infected by HIV are targets of HIV-specific or -nonspecific cellular immune responses which may lead to their elimination by MHC-restricted or -nonrestricted mechanisms [23, 38, 45, 48]. The mechanisms may also include antibody-dependent cellular cytotoxicity (ADCC) [34]. Furthermore, it has been shown that gp120-coated CD4-positive cells are destroyed by natural killer cell-like activity [49].

Indirect Viral Effects. Further disturbance of the process of T4 cell activation may result from structural similarity of viral proteins and proteins that mediate crucial functions of the immune system. The interference of viral protein with ligand-receptor interaction might result in either activation or inhibition of the respective function. Such mechanisms may possibly also contribute to HIV-associated central nervous system damage and impairment of other organ systems. Table 1 shows examples of such mechanisms. By binding to CD4, for example, circulating gp120 may prevent the binding of the natural ligand of CD4, HLA-DR and thus interfere with antigen recognition by T4 cells (see Fig.3). Furthermore, a partial sequence homology of the part of the *env* gene coding for gp120 and of the neuroleukin gene [14] suggests that gp120 may be responsible for the activation of B cells and the secretion of antibodies induced in vitro by lysates of HIV virions [43].

Other examples of sequence or structural homology include $gp120/IgG_{1,2,4}$ and $gp120/IgA_2$ [30], gp41/MHC-II [11], and p17/thymosin α_1 [40].

Induction of Autoimmune Responses by HIV Proteins. The sequence of structural similarity of some viral proteins represents, furthermore, the basis for the induc-

Table 1. Examples of molecular mimicry by HIV-1 which may lead to autoimmunity

HIV protein	Body protein	Area of interference	References
gp120	MHC-II	Antigen recognition by T4 cells	[31, 42]
	Neuroleukin	B-cell activation, neurological functions	[14]
	$IgG_{1,2,4}$ IgA_2	Immune complex formation, rheumatoid factors	[30]
gp41	MHC-II	Antigen recognition by T4 cells	[11]
p17	Thymosin α_1	T-cell activation	[40]

tion of antibodies that may also react with normal body proteins. These antibodies are truly autoimmune in character. Forty percent of patients with AIDS, for example, have antibodies that recognize an HLA-DR derived heptapeptide that possesses a high degree of homology with a heptapeptide of the part of *env* coding for the HIV protein gp41 [11]. These human antibodies may bind to HLA-DR antigens of antigen-presenting cells and thus possibly block the interaction of HLA-DR (MHC-II) with CD4. Similarly, some of the patients' antibodies directed against certain epitopes of gp120 or p17 might interact with their corresponding body proteins and block their function [31, 40, 42]. In addition, autoimmune antibodies have been reported with specificity for proteins that do not have apparent homology with HIV proteins [47].

Tumors in HIV Infection

Recent years have brought several additions to the list of cancers found in association with HIV infection. In addition to KS, NHL, and primary lymphoma of the brain, which are included in the Centers for Disease Control (CDC) definition of AIDS, Hodgkin's lymphoma, oral cancer, rectal carcinoma, testicular cancer, adenosquamous or small-cell carcinoma of the lung (possibly carcinoid), and dermal angiolipoma have been found associated with infection by HIV [1, 13, 16, 29, 50, 51]. Hodgkin's disease in association with HIV infection frequently includes unusual clinical presentations, e.g., involvement of the CNS, the skin, or endobronchial or mesenteric tumors. It is not yet clear whether HIV predisposes to the origin of these tumors or simply modifies the clinical course.

In contrast to the human oncoretroviruses HTLV-I and HTLV-II, HIV does not possess in vitro transforming capacity. HIV provirus is found in none of the tumors associated with AIDS. Therefore its role in tumorigenesis must be indirect. Theoretically, integration of HIV provirus in positions adjacent to cellular oncogenes might lead to their activation, as is the case with chronic animal leukemia viruses. However, such cells are not likely to be resistent to the viral cytopathic effect and would be quickly destroyed. As outlined above, an immunodeficiency as severe as that brought about by HIV infection is sufficient to explain the high incidence of cancer.

Many of the tumors occurring naturally in animals, especially the lmyphomas and leukemias, are associated with retrovirus infection. It is therefore conceivable that some of the tumors now seen in HIV-infected individuals may also be associated with infection by human oncogenic retroviruses. Such viruses would likely have entered and been propagated in the same sexually promiscuous populations now suffering most frequently from the AIDS epidemic. The regionally high incidence of coinfection by the human oncoviruses HTLV-I and HTLV-II in American and European groups at risk for AIDS or in AIDS patients is a good example of this possibility [12, 37]. Concomitant infection with HTLV-I and HIV was reported in a patient with a T8 lymphoproliferative disease [15]. In the future, HTLV-I or -II associated malignant tumors are likely to occur more frequently, but they are not now of quantitative importance.

Infection by DNA viruses is frequently present in groups at risk for AIDS.

Some of these are associated with the development of malignant tumors. These viruses include Epstein-Barr virus (EBV; Burkitt's lymphoma, nasopharyngeal carcinoma, possibly certain thymic lymphomas), hepatitis B virus (hepatocellular carcinoma), cytomegalovirus (CMV; possible association with KS), and human papilloma virus (associated with genital and, possibly, anal carcinoma). Chronic productive infection by these viruses may lead to perpetual growth stimulation of certain target cells which would over time increase the occurrence of mutations that, together with a series of cofactors, finally lead to cancer [21].

The loss of immune surveillance in AIDS may permit activation of latent DNA virus infection, which in turn might induce the pathogenic steps outlined above. In addition, recent results suggest that HIV might act as a promoting factor in DNA virus associated tumors. A related regulatory mechanism of virus expression has been described for HIV, HTLV-I and -II, hepatitis B virus, and members of the papovavirus, adenovirus, and herpesvirus families, including lymphotropic papovaviruses, bovine papilloma virus, CMV, varicella-zoster virus, and herpes simplex viruses. These viruses may trans-activate the LTR-mediated transcription of HIV. Concomitant infection with these viruses is thus likely to promote HIV infection, provided the regulatory proteins of these DNA viruses could enter HIV-infected cells ([9, 32]; R. C. Gallo, communication at the 3rd international conference on AIDS). It is conceivable, although it has not yet been shown, that HIV might in turn act as transcriptional promoter of these viruses.

Kaposi's Sarcoma

KS in AIDS patients is histologically indistinguishable from KS occurring sporadically in older men of Eastern European origin, endemic KS in parts of Central Africa, and KS arising in recipients of organ transplants treated with immunosuppressive drugs. Its rapid progression in HIV-positive patients suggests that both its genesis and its progression are partly influenced by the immune system. A number of other cofactors have also been implicated. CMV was cultured from KS tumors from Africa, and the high prevalence of CMV infection among homosexual men, who are at highest risk to develop KS, suggests a role in its etiology [10]. Other cofactors implicated in HIV-related KS include nitrites and the presence of the HLA-DR5 phenotype [35]. Recently, the incidence of KS in homosexual men with AIDS has been observed to decline, possibly as a consequence of life-style modifications which have reduced CMV infection rates and the use of nitrites [51].

Finally, angiogenic factors may be crucial in the causation of KS. Some cell lines infected by HTLV-II apparently secrete factors which allow the cultivation of KS tumor cells in vitro (R. C. Gallo, communication at the 3rd international congress on AIDS). Hypervascular changes may occur early in lymph nodes of patients with HIV-associated, persistent, generalized lymphadenopathy, then progress to angioimmunoblastic changes, and finally lead to KS [17]. It is possible that HIV infection of certain cells (e.g., monocyte/macophages) may lead to the release of angiogenic materials. A possible model of the pathogenesis of KS is shown in Fig. 4.

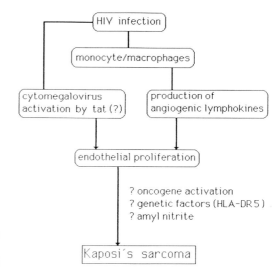

Fig. 4. Possible steps involved in the pathogenesis of HIV-associated Kaposi's sarcoma. (Modified from [51])

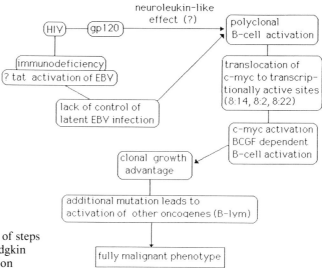

Fig. 5. Possible sequence of steps leading to B-cell non-Hodgkin lymphoma in HIV infection

Non-Hodgkin's Lymphoma in AIDS

NHL of predominately B-cell origin occurs frequently in association with HIV infection. The localization involves uncommon sites, and the course is rapid. The tumors are of monoclonal B-cell origin, have no integrated HIV provirus, but are EBV-positive and show characteristic chromosomal translocations (8:14 q) in most cases studied. Figure 5 shows a possible sequence of pathogenic elements leading to these tumors. B-cell hyperplasia is found early in HIV infection. This may be due partly to EBV activation (possibly also promoted by HIV *trans*-acting factors) and partly to stimulation by a neuroleukin-like effect of gp120 [14, 43]. These mechanisms would lead to polyclonal B-cell activation. According to Klein [21], this condition predisposes to chromosomal injuries resulting in translocation of c-*myc* to transcriptionally active sites such as the immunoglobulin gene loci. Cell clones with such mutations would have a growth advantage which would further increase the chances for mutations. These would lead to activation of additional oncogenes (e.g., *B-lym*) and result in the fully malignant phenotype.

Conclusion

Various types of cancer are associated with abnormalities in the immune system which may include elements of immunodeficiency as well as autoimmunity or chronic inflammation. The frequent occurrence of tumors in typical autoimmune disorders, e.g., Sjögren's disease, sarcoidosis, or pemphigus, is well known. The slowly emerging findings of autoimmune mechanisms in AIDS point to a possibly related etiopathogenesis of such disorders. Recent results suggest that virus groups as distantly related as DNA and RNA viruses may use common regulatory pathways, thus raising the possibility of mutual effects in coinfections. The analysis of HIV disease as a model comprising immunodeficiency, autoimmunity, tumors, and concomitant infection by various agents is difficult, but the effort will lead not only to better treatment and, possibly, prevention of this disease, but also to a better understanding of these other significant disorders.

References

1. Baer DM, Anderson ET, Wilkinson LS (1986) Acquired immune deficiency syndrome in homosexual men with Hodgkin's disease. Am J Med 80: 738–740
2. Barré-Sinoussi F, Chermann JC, Rey F, et al. (1983) Isolation of a T-lymphotropic retrovirus from a patient at risk for acquired immune deficiency syndrome (AIDS). Science 220: 868–871
3. Brun-Vézinet F, Rey MA, Katlama C, et al. (1987) Lymphadenopathy-associated virus type 2 in AIDS and AIDS-related complex. Lancet I: 128–132
4. Clavel F, Guétard D, Brun-Vézinet F, et al. (1986) Isolation of a new human retrovirus from West African patients with AIDS. Science 233: 343–346
5. Clavel F, Mansinho K, Chamaret S, et al. (1987) Human immunodeficiency virus type 2 infection associated with AIDS in West Africa. N Engl J Med 316: 1180–1185
6. Dalgleish AG, Beverley PCL, Clapham PR, et al. (1984) The CD4 (T4) antigen is an essential component of the receptor for the AIDS retrovirus. Nature 312: 763–767
7. Gallo RC, Salahuddin SZ, Popovic M, et al. (1984) Frequent detection and isolation of cytopathic retroviruses (HTLV-III) from patients with AIDS and at risk for AIDS. Science 224: 500–503
8. Gartner SP, Markovits P, Kaplan MH, et al. (1986) The role of mononuclear phagocytes in HTLV-III/LAV infection. Science 233: 215–219
9. Gendelman HE, Phelps W, Feigenbaum L, et al. (1986) Trans-activation of the human immunodeficiency virus long terminal repeat sequence by DNA viruses. Proc Natl Acad Sci USA 83: 9759–9763
10. Giraldo G, Beth E (1986) The involvement of cytomegalovirus in acquired immunodeficiency syndrome. Prog Allergy 37: 319–331

11. Golding H, Robey FA, Gates FT, et al. (1987) Homologous peptides from HIV p41 and HLA class II bind CD4 on human T-cells. 3rd international conference on AIDS, Washington, DC, June 1–5, abstract F.4.2
12. Gradilone A, Zani M, Barillari G, et al. (1986) HTLV-I and HIV in drug addicts in Italy. Lancet II: 753
13. Groopman JE, Mayer K, Zipoli T, et al. (1986) Unusual neoplasms associated with HTLV-III infection. Proc Am Soc Clin Oncol 5: 4
14. Gurney ME, Heinrich SP, Lee MR, Yin H-S (1986) Molecular cloning and expression of neuroleukin, a neurotrophic factor for spinal and sensory neurons. Science 234: 566–573
15. Harper ME, Kaplan MH, Marselle LM, et al. (1986) Concomitant infection with HTLV-I and HTLV-III in a patient with T8 lymphoproliverative disease. N Engl J Med 315: 1073–1078
16. Irwin LE, Begandy MK, Moore TM (1984) Adenosquamous carcinoma of the lung and the acquired immunodeficiency syndrome. Ann Intern Med 100: 158
17. Janossy G, Racz P, Bofill M, et al. (1987) Microenvironmental changes in lymph nodes of homosexual men with HIV infections. In: Gluckman JC, Vilmer E (eds) Acquired immunodeficiency syndrome. Elsevier, Paris, pp 87–96
18. Kanki PJ, Barin F, M'Boup S, et al. (1986) New human T-lymphotropic retrovirus related to simian T-lymphotropic virus type III (STLV-III$_{AGM}$). Science 232: 238–243
19. Klatzmann D, Barré-Sinoussi F, Nugeyre MT et al. (1984a) Selective tropism of lymphadenopathy associated virus (LAV) for helper-inducer T-lymphocytes. Science 225: 59–63
20. Klatzmann D, Champagne E, Chamaret S, et al. (1984b) T-lymphocyte T4 molecule behaves as the receptor for human retrovirus LAV. Nature 312: 767–768
21. Klein G (1986) Evolution of tumors and the impact of molecular oncology. Nature 315: 190–195
22. Koenig S, Gendelman HE, Orenstein JM, et al. (1986) Detection of AIDS virus in macrophages in brain tissue from AIDS patients with encephalopathy. Science 233: 1089–1093
23. Koenig S, Earl P, Powell D, et al. (1987) Cytotoxic T-cells directed against target cells expressing HIV-1 proteins. 3rd international conference of AIDS, Washington DC, June 1–5, abstract T.9.3
24. Kreiss JK, Koech D, Plummer FA, et al. (1986) AIDS virus infection in Nairobi prostitutes – Spread of the epidemic to East Africa. N Engl J Med 314: 414–418
25. Lane HC, Depper JM, Greene WC, et al. (1985) Qualitative analysis of immune function in patients with the acquired immunodeficiency syndrome: evidence for a selective defect in soluble antigen recognition. N Engl J Med 313: 79–84
26. Levy JA, Hoffmann AD, Kramer SM, et al. (1984) Isolation of lymphocytopathic retroviruses from San Francisco patients with AIDS. Science 225: 840–842
27. Levy JA, Shimabukuro J, McHugh T, et al. (1985) AIDS-associated retroviruses (ARV) can productively infect other cells besides human T helper cells. Virology 147: 441–448
28. Lifson JD, Reyes GR, McGratz MS, et al. (1986) AIDS retrovirus induced cytopathology: giant cell formation and involvement of CD4 antigen. Science 232: 1123–1127
29. Lozada F, Silverman S, Conant M (1982) New outbreak of oral tumors, malignancies and infectious diseases strikes young male homosexuals. Calif Dent J 10: 39–42
30. Maddon PJ, Dalgleish AG, McDougal JS, et al. (1986) The T4 gene encodes the AIDS virus receptor and is expressed in the immune system and the brain. Cell 47: 333–348
31. Montagnier L, Gruest J, Klatzmann D, Gluckmann JC (1986) Anti-class II monoclonal antibodies inhibit LAV infection of CEM cells. International conference on AIDS, Paris, June 22–24, abstract 261
32. Mosca JD, Bednarik DP, Raj NBK, et al. (1987) Herpes simplex virus type 1 can reactivate transcription of latent human immunodeficiency virus. Nature 325: 67–70

33. Nicholson JKA, Cross GD, Callaway CS, McDougal JS (1986) In vitro infection of human monocytes with human T lymphotropic virus type III/lymphadenopathy-associated virus (HTLV-III/LAV). J Immunol 137: 323-328

34. Ojo-Amaize E, Nishanian PG, Keith D, et al. (1987) HIV antibodies in human sera induce cell-mediated lysis of HIV-infected cells. 3rd international conference on AIDS, Washington DC, June 1-5, abstract T.9.6

35. Pollack MS, Falk J, Gazit E, et al. (1984) Classical and AIDS-Kaposi's sarcoma. In: Albert ED, Baur MP, Mayr WR (eds) Histocompatibility testing 1984. Springer, Berlin Heidelberg New York, pp 403-406

36. Popovic M, Sarngadharan MG, Read E, Gallo RC (1984) Detection, isolation, and continuous production of cytopathic retroviruses (HTLV-III) from patients with AIDS and pre-AIDS. Science 224: 497-500

37. Robert-Guroff M, Blayney DW, Safai B, et al. (1984) HTLV-I-specific antibody in AIDS patients and others at risk. Lancet II: 128-130

38. Ruscetti FW, Mikovits JA, Kalyanaraman VS, et al. (1986) Analysis of effector mechanisms against HTLV-I- and HTLV-III/LAV-infected lymphoid cells. J Immunol 136: 3619-3624

39. Safai G, Koziner B (1965) Malignant neoplasms in AIDS. In: DeVita VT Jr, Hellman S, Rosenberg SA (eds) AIDS - etiology, diagnosis, treatment and prevention. Lippincott, Philadelphia, pp 213-222

40. Sarin PS, Sun DK, Thornton AH, et al. (1986) Neutralization of HTLV-III/LAV replication by antiserum to thymosin-alpha$_1$. Science 232: 1135-1137

41. Sarngadharan MG, Popovic M, Bruch L, et al. (1984) Antibodies reactive with human T-lymphotropic retroviruses (HTLV-III) in the serum of patients with AIDS. Science 224: 506-508

42. Sattentau QJ, Dalgleish A, Beverley PCL, Weiss R (1986) Epitopes of the CD4 (T4) molecule and HTLV-III infection. International conference on AIDS, Paris, June 23-25, abstract 159

43. Schnittman SM, Lance HC, Higgins SE, et al. (1986) Direct polyclonal activation of human B lymphocytes by the acquired immune deficiency syndrome virus. Science 233: 1084-1086

44. Schüpbach J, Popovic M, Gilden RV, et al. (1984) Serological analysis of a subgroup of human T-lymphotropic retroviruses (HTLV-III) associated with AIDS. Science 224: 503-505

45. Shepp DH, Mann D, Chakrabarti S, et al. (1987) Detection of HLA restricted human immunodeficiency virus (HIV) envelope antigen-specific cytotoxic lymphocytes (CTL). 3rd international conference on AIDS, Washington DC, June 1-5, abstract T.9.2

46. Sodroski J, Goh WC, Rosen C, et al. (1986) Role of the HTLV-III/LAV envelope in syncytium formation and cytopathicity. Nature 322: 470-474

47. Stricker RB, McHug TM, Moody DJ, et al. (1987) An AIDS-related cytotoxic autoantibody reacts with a specific antigen on stimulated CD4$^+$ cells. Nature 327: 710-713

48. Walker BD, Chakrabarti S, Moss B, et al. (1987) HIV env- and gag-specific cytotoxic T lymphocytes (CTL's) in seropositive individuals. 3rd international conference on AIDS, Washington DC, June 1-5, abstract T.9.1

49. Weinhold KJ, Lyerly HK, Mattews TJ, et al. (1987) Gp120-specific cell-mediated cytotoxicity in patients exposed to HIV. 3rd international conference on AIDS, Washington DC, June 1-5, abstract T.9.4

50. Weldon-Linne CM, Rhone DP, Blatt D, et al. (1984) Angiolipomas in homosexual men. N Engl J Med 310: 1193-1194

51. Ziegler JL (1987) AIDS and cancer. In: Gluckman JC, Vilmer E (eds) Acquired immunodeficiency syndrome. Elsevier, Paris, pp 219-226

52. Schüpbach J (1987) AIDS Antigen/Antikörpersysteme im Kontext des Immunsystems. In: Siegenthaler W (ed) Aktuelle Aspekte der Infektiologie. 19.Symposium der Gesellschaft für Fortschritte auf dem Gebiet der Inneren Medizin. Thieme, Stuttgart, pp 19-31

Immunological Characteristics and Potential Approaches to Immunotherapy of HIV Infection

E. M. Hersh, E. A. Petersen, D. E. Yocum, S. R. Gorman, M. J. Darragh, C. R. Gschwind, G. W. Brewton, and J. A. Reuben

Section of Hematology and Oncology, Department of Internal Medicine, University of Arizona Health Science Center, Tucson, AZ 85724, USA

Many of the immunological mechanisms associated with the development and pathogenesis of AIDS are now well understood [10]. Thus, T-cell activation and proliferation facilitate HIV infection and virus proliferation. Macrophages, B cells, endothelial cells, and brain cells may also become infected. T-cell depletion resulting from lysis, syncytium formation, and anti-T-cell autoantibody is the fundamental immunological defect. Neutralizing antibody to virus-membrane antigens may play an important role in prognosis. Pathogenesis is related, in part, to the activity of cofactors such as Epstein-Barr virus EBV and cytomegalovirus CMV infection. Immunological mechanisms in HIV infection are summarized in Fig. 1. Chronic active infections in intravenous drug abusers and homosexuals are important contributing factors. This can itself result in immunodeficiency, which has been demonstrated in EBV, CMV, herpes simplex virus (HSV), and hepatitis B infections. It can also result in chronic antigenic stimulation and immune activation. The latter can also be seen in hemophiliacs, secondary to chronic blood product administration. Surgically induced stress followed by transfusion of HIV-contaminated blood is also important. The immune activation and immune deficiency produced by the above allow for facilitation of the HIV infection. Once infection is established, progression of disease, CD4-positive cell depletion, and

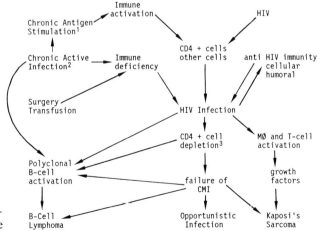

Fig. 1. Immunological mechanisms in HIV infection; [1] hemophilia; [2] Epstein-Barr virus, cytomegalovirus, herpes simplex virus, hepatitis B; [3] lysis, syncytium formation, autoantibody; *M0*, macrophage

other manifestations such as macrophage and T-cell activation or polyclonal B-cell activation depend upon the balance between the immune-activating, immunodeficiency-producing, and specific anti-HIV immunity factors. Ultimately, polyclonal B-cell activation will result in B-cell lymphoma, and CD4-positive cell depletion will result in a failure of cell-mediated immunity and opportunistic infection, while the failure of cell-mediated immunity combined with growth factors produced during the above process may result in Kaposi's sarcoma.

The serologic relationship between HIV and EBV infection in HIV-infected subjects has been demonstrated by Rinaldo and coworkers [14]. They have shown a correlation between the antibody titer to HIV and rising antibody titers to EBV capsid and EBV early antigen, while there was no relationship to CMV or HSV antibody titers. This is an example of how cofactors interact with HIV to produce both immunodeficiency and one of the AIDS-related complications (EBV-induced malignant lymphoma).

Table 1 summarizes immunological and related abnormalities associated with HIV infection. Clinically, there are autoimmune and inflammatory diseases, such as idiopathic thrombocytopenic purpura (ITP), psoriasis, and an increased incidence of certain allergies, such as those to sulfonamides. The immunodeficiency results in anergy to recall skin-test antigens as well as opportunistic infections and malignancy. Circulating interferons and immune complexes are detected and are associated with a poor prognosis.

Leukocyte counts are often abnormal and include lymphopenia, CD4-positive cell depletion, and inversion of the CD4/CD8 ratio at an early stage. Later there may be granulocytopenia monocytopenia, and thrombocytopenia resulting from myelodysplastic changes in the bone marrow.

Serologically, these patients are characterized by hypergammaglobulinemia. At least among the homosexual and intravenous drug abuser groups, seropositivity to CMV, EBV, and hepatitis B are present in virtually 100% of patients. More recently, autoantibodies to T cells have been discovered and have been implicated as a significant cause of the T-cell depletion in these patients. In addition, the presence of acid-labile α-Interferon, β_2-microglobulin, and immune complexes in the serum are poor prognostic signs. The T-cell depletion as well as perturbed function of residual T cells (which we have shown is related to augmented supressor-cell activity) is responsible for a wide variety of abnormal immune functions, including impaired mitogen responses to T-cell and T-dependent B-cell mitogens, impaired allogeneic mixed lymphocyte reaction (MLR) and autologous MLR, impaired proliferative responses to microbial antigens including viral antigens, impaired interferon and interleukin production, and impaired natural killer (NK) cell and cytotoxic T-lymphocyte (CTL) activity and antibody dependent cell-mediated cytotoxicity (ADCC). In addition, T-cell help to B-cell responses is impaired. While it has not received a great deal of attention, macrophage-related immunodysregulation has also been noted [2]. Immunodysregulation is characteristic of this disease, and it includes hypergammaglobulinemia, the development of autoantibodies, the presence of circulating immune complexes, and impaired primary and possibly secondary antibody responses.

The serology of AIDS is important [15]. Shortly after infection, patients develop antibody to gp41 and gp120 cell-membrane antigens as well as to internal antigens

Table 1. Immunological and related abnormalities associated with HIV infection

Clinical
  Autoimmune disease (ITP)
  Inflammatory disease (psoriasis-like)
  Increased allergy (sulfonamides)
  Immunodeficiency
    Skin-test anergy (delayed hypersensitivity)
    Opportunistic infection
    Opportunistic malignancy
  Circulating interferon
  Circulating immune complexes

Laboratory
  Leukocytes
    Lymphopenia
    CD4 + cell depletion
    Inverted CD4/CD8 ratio
    Other lymphocyte subset abnormalities
    Granulocytopenia
    Monocytopenia
    Thrombocytopenia
  Marrow
    Myelodysplastic syndrome
  Serum
    Hypergammaglobulinemia
    Seropositivity: HIV, CMV, EBV, hepatitis B
    Autoanti-T-cell antibody
    Acid-labile α-interferon
    β_2-Microglobulin
    Immune complexes

T-cell-related immunodeficiency
  T-cell mitogen responses: PHA, CON-A
  T-dependent B-cell mitogen responses: pokeweed mitogen
  Allogeneic MLR
  Autologous MLR
  Proliferative responses to microbial antigens
  Interferon production
  Interleukin 2 production and response
  NK and CTL activity, ADCC
  T-cell help to B-cell response

Macrophage-related immunodysregulation
  Monocyte adherence
  Interferon and other cytokine production
  Monocyte-suppressor activity
  Monocyte-mediated cytotoxicity

B-cell-related dysregulation
  Hypergammaglobulinemia
  Autoantibodies
  Circulating immune complexes
  Impaired primary and possibly secondary antibody responses

Table 2. Immunological factors relating to stage and/or prognosis in HIV-infected patients

Stage
  Delayed hypersensitivity
  T-cell and T-cell subset numbers
  CD4/CD8 ratio
  Mitogen, MLR and antigen responses
  NK, ADCC, and CTL responses
  Serum interferon
  Serum β_2-microglobulin
  Serum-immune complexes
  Anti-p24 antibody

Prognosis
  Absolute blood level of CD4 + lymphocytes
  CD4/CD8 ratio
  Delayed hypersensitivity to recall antigens
  Proliferative response to mitogen or antigen
  Immune complexes
  Serum interferon

such as p24, p17, etc. As long as the patient remains asymptomatic, these antibodies persist. Upon the development of symptomatic AIDS or AIDS-related complex (ARC) patients usually lose anti-p24, while showing a persistence of anti-gp41 and gp120. At the same time immune complexes appear. Recently, it has been shown that the persistence of high titers of neutralizing antibody is associated with a good prognosis, and that loss of neutralizing antibody is associated with a poor prognosis [5].

A variety of cellular immunological factors are related to stage and/or prognosis in HIV-infected patients; these are shown in Table 2. Probably the most important for both are delayed-type hypersensitivity, the absolute levels of total T cells and the helper T-cell subset, and the CD-4/CD8 ratio. There is some controversy over these features. For example, Abrams [1] found that the most important prognostic variables for progression from the lymphadenopathy syndrome to AIDS were antecedent thrush, elevated erythrocyte sedimentation rate, thrombocytopenia and leukopenia – and not the above-mentioned parameters. In contrast, Vadhan-Raj et al. [17] found the prognosis of patients with Kaposi's sarcoma (regarding remission rate and development of opportunistic infection) to be related to delayed hypersensitivity, total mature T-cell numbers, lymphocyte-proliferative responses to phytohemagglutin (PHA) and *Escherichia coli* antigen and circulating serum interferon. However, in a similar study, Taylor and coworkers [16] found that in Kaposi's sarcoma the most important prognostic variables were the CD4/CD8 ratio and the absolute number of CD4-positive cells, while other parameters were not prognostic. In our own studies [7] we found highly significant correlations between stage of disease (symptom-free, ARC, or AIDS) and a wide variety of immunological parameters (Table 3).

A variety of additional studies shed further light on the immunological status. For example, we and others have demonstrated that patients with ARC and

Table 3. Relationship of host defense parameter to stage of disease in patients with HIV infection

Parameter	Normal	HIV-infected		
		Symptom-free	ARC	AIDS
Abs. lymphocyte count[a]	2.3	1.7	1.8	1.4
Abs. T11 + cell count[a]	1.6	1.5	1.6	1.1
Abs. T3 + cell count[a]	1.7	1.3	1.5	0.85
Abs. T4 + cell count[a]	1.0	0.6	0.65	0.35
Abs. T8 + cell count[a]	0.63	0.62	0.81	0.63
Natural killer cell activity[b]	19.1	4.5	16.8	12.5
PHA response[c]	114.4	76.4	82.5	78.9
Pokeweed mitogen response[c]	50.6	40.9	36.9	21.1
CON-A response[c]	68.6	36.7	45.2	22.2
Monocyte adherence[d]	15.9	12.6	9.1	4.8
Serum lysozyme[e]	7.4	9.1	13.2	10.5
Number of positive delayed-hypersensitivity skin tests per seven applied	4.1	1.8	1.8	0.8

All patient parameters showed significant reduction compared to normal except for absolute (Abs.) T8 + cell count. In addition, there was a significant progressive reduction in parameters within the patient groups comparing the symptom-free to those with ARC and AIDS.

[a] Cells/mm^3 $\times$ 10^{-3}.
[b] Percent target lysis.
[c] cpm/culture $\times$ 10^{-3}.
[d] Adherent monocytes/ml blood $\times$ 10^{-4}.
[e] μg/ml.

AIDS, as well as asymptomatic HIV-infected subjects, have markedly impaired in vitro responses to HSV and CMV [6]. This includes lymphocyte proliferation, NK-cell activation, and interferon production. Thus, a vicious circle is established: T-cell immunodeficiency augments these viral infections which, in turn, can worsen immunodeficiency. In a second study, we demonstrated markedly augmented suppressor-cell activity in patients with ARC and AIDS [8]. In this study, normal lymphocytes were cocultured with patient lymphocytes, which resulted in an abrogation of the normal lymphocyte-proliferative responses to mitogens. If the patient's cells were irradiated, this supressor-cell activity was abolished. This suggests that there is intrinsic T helper cell deficiency, and in addition that the residual helper cells are suppressed by activated supressor cells.

An area of growing importance is that of the careful study of anti-HIV immunity. Humoral immunity has already been discussed above. Cellular immunity would include cell-mediated cytotoxicity, such as NK, CTL, and macrophage-mediated reactivity against HIV-infected cells as well as ADCC to infected cells. Furthermore, it would involve proliferative responses to virus-infected cells or membrane preparations and to viral antigens themselves. We have begun preliminary

Table 4. Cytotoxicity of peripheral blood mononuclear cells from HIV-infected asymptomatic and early ARC patients to various target cell lines

Target cell	Effector cell processing	Serum	E:T ratio	Percent cytotoxicity	
				Patient cells	Normal cells
K562	–	FCS	5:1	10.5	16.0
K562	–	FCS	25:1	31.0	37.5
Daudi	–	FCS	5:1	2.0	2.0
Daudi	–	FCS	25:1	6.0	5.0
Daudi	IL-2, 3 days	FCS	25:1	72.5	73.0
CR10	–	FCS	25:1	6.5	4.1
CR10	–	α HIV (patient)	25:1	18.4	13.1
CR10	IL-2, 4 h	FCS	25:1	26.0	32.0
CR10	IL-2, 3 h	FCS	25:1	43.5	43.0

K562, erythroleukemia cell line, NK cell target; *Daudi,* Burkitt's lymphoma B-cell line; *CR10,* HIV-infected CEM cell line; *FCS,* fetal calf serum; *IL-2,* interleukin-2 incubated with effector cells 3 days or 4 h before cytotoxicity assay; *α HIV* (patient), patient serum with anti-gp41 and gp120 activity. All assays were conducted by a standard 4-h chromium-release method. Values shown are medians.

experiments along these lines, which are summarized in Table 4. We have focused on patients with asymptomatic HIV infection or with early ARC, thinking that these would manifest the greatest anti-HIV immunity and would be most susceptible to immunomodulation therapy. As shown, we have found that NK cell reactivity to K562 is normal in these patients, and that by in vitro incubation with interleukin 2 their peripheral blood mononuclear cells can be induced to high cytolytic activity against Daudi cells.

Furthermore, we have used the HIV-infected CEM cell line (CR-10) (obtained from Dr. David Volsky of the University of Nebraska) to study the cytotoxicity of peripheral blood mononuclear cells of patients against a relevant target. Neither patients nor normals lysed CEM CR-10 well in fetal calf serum, but when the cells were preincubated with patient serum, lysis was observed (somewhat higher in the patients than in the normals). Furthermore, in the presence of interleukin 2 either for 4 h or 3 days, significantly augmented lysis occurred. Thus, immunomodulation may augment specific anti-HIV cell-mediated cytolysis. Several investigators have attempted to use genetically engineered HIV antigens as lymphocyte stimulants. In vitro responses have not been seen. The explanation for this is not clear, but it may provide a clue to specific cellular immunodeficiency in this disease.

With this immunological background, it is appropriate to consider the immunotherapy of AIDS. Discussion of a preventive vaccine is beyond the scope of this review. We will focus on immunorestorative and immunomodulatory therapy, either alone or in combination with non-immunological approaches. Approaches to immunotherapy are summarized in Table 5.

Table 5. Immunotherapeutic approaches to HIV infection

Immunorestoration
Natural
  Thymic hormones
  Transfer factors
  Tuftsin
  Cytokines
    γ-Interferon
    Interleukin 2
    Interleukin 4
Synthetic
  Imuthiol
  Isoprinosine
  Azimexon

Immunomodulation
Antisuppressor T-cell
Anti-suppressor macrophage

Active immunotherapy
Nonspecific macrophage activation
  Granulocyte macrophage colony-stimulating factor
  Muramyl tripeptide analogue
Active-specific immunization against HIV or HIV antigens
  Cellular immunity
  Humoral immunity

Passive and serotherapy
Nonspecific γ-globulin
Specific anti-HIV antibody
Removal of immune complexes plasma immunoabsorption

Bone marrow transplantation

The immunorestorative drug diethyldithiocarbamate (DTC), or imuthiol, has been of special interest to us. In animal systems this agent is immunorestorative in immunodeficient aged mice, chemotherapy- and radiotherapy-treated mice, nude mice, and New Zealand black mice [13]. Several positive clinical trials with DTC in AIDS have already been reported in each, the benefits were more prominent in ARC than in AIDS. The findings include amelioration of AIDS-related symptoms, reduction in lymphadenopathy, improvement in immunological parameters, elimination of some specific AIDS-related manifestations such as hairy leukoplakia and ITP, and diminished progression of disease. We are currently conducting a randomized dose-response study of DTC in ARC and AIDS patients [9]. Doses from 200 to 800 mg/m^2 once or twice weekly are being explored. The findings in this ongoing study include diminished symptomatology, reduced lymph node size, improved immunological parameters, and diminished progression (Table 6). DTC is also being explored in an animal model. We have used the LPBM-5 retrovirus model of AIDS in the mouse [12]. Infected mice develop lymphadenopathy, polyclonal B-cell activation, hypergammaglobulinemia, T-cell immunodeficiency, late opportunistic infections, and neurological complications. In our preliminary

Table 6. Preliminary results of diethyldithiocarbamate therapy in patients with ARC and AIDS

Parameters	Treated ($n = 10$)		Control ($n = 11$)	
	pre	post	pre	post
Average number or symptoms per patient	2.1	1.3	1.5	1.7
Average number of nodes per patient	3.4	1.6	3.5	3.5
Sum median node diameter (cm)	10.0	6.6	13.3	12.0
Lymphocyte count (cells/mm$^3 \times 10^{-3}$)	0.99	1.6	1.2	0.87
CD4 + cell count (cells/mm$^3 \times 10^{-3}$)	0.08	0.26	0.05	0.08
Progressors		3 (30%)		7 (64%)
Alive		9 (90%)		8 (73%)

Table 7. Effects of diethyldithiocarbamate *(DTC)* on the LPBM5 retrovirus-induced immunocysregulation in C57 BL mice

Host parameter	Virus infected	DTC--treated	Host parameter measurement on day		
			15	42	63
Serum IgM (mg/ml)	−	−	0.8	0.9	1.3
	+	−	0.9	7.9	9.3
	+	+	0.6	2.7	6.3
PHA (cpm $\times 10^{-3}$)	−	−	141	101	86
	+	−	32	5	3
	+	+	57	18	16
Lipopolysaccharide (cpm $\times 10^{-3}$)	−	−	135	143	140
	+	−	69	28	12
	+	+	41	42	58
Spleen weight (gm)	−	−	−	0.10	−
	+	−	−	0.40	−
	+	+	−	0.17	−

Days refers to day after virus innoculation.

studies in this model (Table 7) we have found that DTC reduces hypergammaglobulinemia, reduces spleen weight, and partially maintains T-cell and B-cell immunocompetence compared to untreated controls. This model provides an ideal setting in which to study immunorestorative drugs and their combination with other therapies such as antiretroviral therapy.

Finally, we have an interesting anecdote bearing on the above (Fig. 2). We have treated a patient with Hodgkin's disease in remission after extensive chemotherapy and radiotherapy who suffered from severe immunodeficiency, repeated opportunistic viral and bacterial infections, and severe malaise. After treatment with DTC, at 200 mg/m^2 weekly, the malaise and opportunistic infection disappeared in association with restoration of normal immunocompetence.

From all of the above, a strategy for clinical research on the immunological approaches to AIDS therapy can be developed. First, we recommend that patients

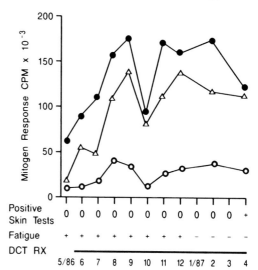

Fig. 2. Effect of diethyldithiocarbamate *(DTC)* therapy on the clinical and immunological status of a patient with Hodgkin's disease. *Open circles,* pokeweed mitogen; *filled circles,* phytohemagglutinin; *open triangles,* concanavalin-A

with HIV infection be treated as early as possible with long-term nontoxic therapy encompassing both antivirals and immunorestoratives. In addition, when HSV, CMV, or EBV infection is present (as manifested serologically), careful consideration should be given to intermittent or continuous therapy directed against these cofactor viruses. Of course, the same applies to patients with ARC and AIDS, but they are less likely to respond or their response will be more difficult to evaluate. However, they certainly are candidates for experimental therapy of this type. Finally, specific immunotherapy directed against HIV should be considered. Thus, active immunization with immunogenic HIV antigen preparations might result in the development of both cellular and humoral immunity to HIV, which would be effective in eliminating or reducing the level of the virus as well as the number of virus-infected cells. Finally, as human monoclonal antibody technology develops, it certainly should be possible to develop neutralizing, human IgG-type anti-HIV antibodies. These should also be studied for their potential to reduce virus infection within patients, therefore improving their prognosis.

References

1. Abrams DI (1986) Lymphadenopathy related to the acquired immunodeficiency syndrome in homosexual men. Med Clin North Am 70: 693–706
2. Braun DP, Harris JE (1986) Abnormal monocyte function in patients with Kaposi's Sarcoma. Cancer 57: 1501–1506
3. Brewton GW, Hersh EM, Mansell P, Rios A, Reuben J (1987) Use of Imuthiol[1] (Diethyldithiocarbamate, DTC) in symptomatic HIV infection. 3rd international conference on AIDS, Washington DC, June 1–5, p 49
4. Caraux J et al. (1987) Treatment of ARC patients with sodium Diethyldithiocarbamate (DTC-Imuthiol) a multicentric, randomized, placebo-controlled trial. 3rd international conference on AIDS, Washington DC, June 1–5, p 49

5. Faulkner-Valle GP, De-Rossi A, Dalla-Gassa O, Chieco-Bianchi L (1986) LAV/HTLV-III neutralizing antibodies in the sera of patients with AIDS, Lymphadenopathy syndrome and asymptomatic seropositive individuals. Tumori 72: 219–224

6. Hersh EM, Gutterman JU, Spector S, et al. (1985) Impaired in vitro interferon, blastogenic, and natural killer cell responses to viral stimulation in acquired immune deficiency syndrome. Cancer Res 45: 406–410

7. Hersh EM, Mansell PWA, Reuben JM, et al. (1984) Immunological characterization of patients with AIDS, the AIDS-related symptom complex and an AIDS-related life style. Cancer Res 44: 5894–5901

8. Hersh EM, Mansell PWA, Reuben JM, et al. (1983) Supressor cell activity among the peripheral blood leukocytes of homosexual patients. Cancer 43: 1905–1909

9. Hersh EM, Petersen E, Yocum DE, Gorman RS, Darragh JM (1987) Dose response study of diethyldithiocarbamate (DTC or Imuthiol) in patients with ARC and AIDS. Proc Am Soc Clin Oncol 6: 2

10. Lang W, Anderson RE, Perkins H, et al. (1985) Clinical, immunologic, and serologic findings in men at risk for acquired immunodeficiency syndrome. JAMA 257: 326–330

11. Lange JM, Oberling F, Aleksyevic A, et al. (1985) Immunomodulation with diethyldithiocarbamate in patients with AIDS-related complex. Lancet 2: 1066

12. Mosier DE, Yetter RA, Morse HC III (1985) J Exp Med 161: 766

13. Renoux G, Renoux M (1977) Thymus-like activities of sulphur derivatives in T-cell differenciation. J Exp Med 145 (2): 466–471

14. Rinaldo CR JR, Kingsley LA, Lyter DW, Rabin BS, Atchison RW, Bodner AJ, Weiss SH, Saxinger WC (1986) Association of HTLV-III with Epstein-Barr virus infection and abnormalities of T Lymphocytes in homosexual men. J Infect Dis 154: 556–561

15. Sarngadharan MG, Popovic M, Bruch L, et al. (1984) Antibodies reactive with human T-lymphotropic retroviruses (HTLV-III) in the serum of patients with AIDS. Science 224: 506–508

16. Taylor J, Afrasiabi R, Fahey JL, Korns E, Weaver M, Mitsuyasu R (1986) Prognostically significant classification of immune changes in AIDS with Kaposi's sarcoma. Blood 67: 666–671

17. Vadhan-Raj S, Wong G, Gnecco C, Cunningham-Rundles S, Krim M, Real FX, Oettgen HF, Krown SE (1986) Immunological variables as predictors of prognosis in patients with Kaposi's Sarcoma and the acquired immunodeficiency syndrome. Cancer Res 46: 417–425

AIDS-Related Kaposi's Sarcoma*

A. E. Friedman-Kien

Department of Dermatology and Microbiology, New York University Medical Center, 550 First Avenue, New York, NY 10016, USA

Recognition of a New Epidemic

An unusually disseminated, aggressive form of Kaposi's sarcoma and *Pneumocystis carinii* pneumonia, a rare "opportunistic" infection, have remained, respectively, the most frequently observed neoplastic and infectious manifestations of the acquired immune deficiency syndrome (AIDS) in the United States and Europe since the beginning of the epidemic [1, 2]. Twenty-six cases of what is now known as AIDS-associated Kaposi's sarcoma were first seen in homosexual and bisexual men in New York City and California between November 1979 and April 1981 [3]. At the same time in Los Angeles five cases of *P. carinii* pneumonia were also reported in young homosexual men [1]. Kaposi's sarcoma, *P. carinii* pneumonia, and other live-threatening opportunistic infections were previously known to occur in association with diseases involving defective cell-mediated immunity as seen in patients with congenital immunodeficiencies, lymphoreticular malignancies, renal transplant recipients, and other patients receiving immunosuppressive therapy [4]. The sudden epidemic occurrence of Kaposi's sarcoma and unusual opportunistic infections among previously "healthy" individuals who had no recognizable cause of immunosuppression suggested a common, underlying acquired immunologic disorder and eventually led to the realization that a new epidemic, now called AIDS, was on the horizon. Within a few months similar cases were seen among intravenous drug abusers and eventually in hemophiliacs and other recipients of blood products and blood transfusions. Over the next few years heterosexual partners of individuals with AIDS and infants born to mothers with AIDS also developed the syndrome.

The cause of the profound and irreversible underlying immune disorder characteristic of AIDS is believed to be due to a human RNA retrovirus, first isolated in 1982–1983. It was originally known as human T-cell lymphotropic virus type III (HTLV-III) or lymphadenopathy-associated virus (LAV-1) but is now referred to as the human immunodeficiency virus (HIV). Like hepatitis B virus, HIV is blood-borne and sexually transmitted [5].

---

* This research was supported by the Howard Gilman Foundation and the Samuel and May Rudin Foundation, both of New York.

Kaposi's sarcoma was initially described in 1872 by Morictz Kaposi, a Viennese professor of dermatology, as "idiopathic multiple pigmented sarcoma tumors of the skin on the lower extremities" seen in three adult males of Eastern European origin [6]. The red to purple tumors of Kaposi's sarcoma are believed to arise from endothelial cells that line the lymphatics and blood vessels of the skin and, less commonly, other organs [4]. The originally described, relatively benign form of this neoplasm, referred to as "classical" Kaposi's sarcoma, is predominantly seen in elderly men between 50 and 80 years of age (male to female ratio of 10 or 15 to 1) and tends to run an indolent course of 10-15 years. In the 1950s a more aggressive form of Kaposi's sarcoma was found to be one of the most common and endemic tumors seen in equatorial Africa, observed mostly in black adult males 25-40 years of age [7]. A very rare lymphadenopathic form of Kaposi's sarcoma is also found in Africa, primarily seen in young children [8]. In the 1960s patients with kidney transplants and other individuals receiving iatrogenic immunosuppressive therapy were also found to develop Kaposi's sarcoma [9].

In contrast to the classical and the endemic varieties of African Kaposi's sarcoma, patients with AIDS-related Kaposi's sarcoma have primarily been young homosexual men ranging in age from 19 to 64, with a mean age of 37.7 years (W. Meade Morgan, CDC, AIDS Branch, Division of Biostatics; personal communication, 1987). The AIDS-related, fulminant variant of this tumor, referred to as epidemic Kaposi's sarcoma, behaves in a rapidly aggressive manner and is often widely disseminated.

Breakdown of Risk Groups

Homosexual and bisexual men have accounted for about 73 % of the total number of persons with AIDS in the United States. Other populations have also been found to be at increased risk for AIDS, including heterosexual male and female intravenous drug abusers (17%) who are known to share HIV-infected needles and syringes, hemophiliacs (1%) who have received HIV-infected factor VIII clotting concentrates, recipients of HIV-contaminated blood transfusions or blood products (2%), heterosexual partners of HIV-infected individuals (3%), and infants born to HIV-infected mothers (1%). For the remaining 3 % of reported cases of AIDS in the United States, none of the recognized risk factors have been determined [4].

One of the most remarkable and perplexing aspects of this disease is that 95 % of all cases of AIDS-associated Kaposi's sarcoma seen in the United States have been, and continue to be, diagnosed among homosexual AIDS patients [4]. The remaining 5% of all AIDS-associated Kaposi's sarcoma cases in the United States have been reported among heterosexual men and women from the other populations now identified as high-risk groups for AIDS. Of these groups, only 3% of male and female intravenous drug users with AIDS have developed Kaposi's sarcoma; 3.5% of transfusion recipients; 1.5% of hemophiliacs 1.9% of heterosexual contacts of individuals at known risk; 8.5% of individuals born in Haiti or central Africa where most AIDS cases have as of yet no identified risk; and 9.1% of patients with no identified risk factors for AIDS. In addition, there have been

11 cases of Kaposi's sarcoma reported among the 527 children with AIDS (2.1%) in the United States. Almost all of these children had parents who either had AIDS or were known to be members of typical risk groups for AIDS (statistical breakdown supplied by the Center for Disease Control, July 13, 1987).

Since the first recognition of the AIDS epidemic the incidence of Kaposi's sarcoma among homosexual men with AIDS in the United States has steadily decreased from about 44% in 1981 to approximately 20% in 1987 among all patients with AIDS (95% of Kaposi's sarcoma is still seen among homosexual patients). Among the possible reasons suggested for the declining incidence of AIDS-associated Kaposi's sarcoma are changes in high-risk sexual behavior such as anal intercourse among homosexuals, fewer numbers of sexual partners, and reduction in the use of recreational drugs such as butyl or amyl nitrites among this risk group [4]. The decrease in the frequency of AIDS-related Kaposi's sarcoma may also be due to inaccurate reporting to the Centers for Disease Control (CDC). Although the CDC epidemiologic records have been collected in the same manner since 1981, it is possible that many physicians make the diagnosis of Kaposi's sarcoma on clinical grounds without performing tissue biopsies; such cases may not be reported to the CDC. There are also many cases of Kaposi's sarcoma that develop later in the course of a previously diagnosed AIDS patient's illness, following one or more opportunistic infections, which are also not reported and therefore may not be included in the more recent epidemiologic statistics [10].

Diagnosis

The chance discovery of one or more asymptomatic skin lesions of Kaposi's sarcoma is often the first and only hallmark of AIDS seen in an otherwise "healthy" individual. Physicians are now aware of frequently observed early clinical signs of any immunodeficiency due to HIV infection (referred to as AIDS-related complex, ARC), including the development of one or more symptoms such as persistent lymphadenopathy, oral candidiasis (thrush), oral "hairy" leukoplakia, unexplained weight loss, malaise, fatigue, intermittent fevers, drenching "night sweats", diarrhea, and a mild unproductive cough [11].

The occurence or the more serious manifestations of AIDS, life-threatening opportunistic infections such as *carinii* pneumonia, cryptococcosis, toxoplasmosis, tuberculosis and the development of HIV-related neurologic diseases such as dementia or non-Hodgkin's lymphomas confer a grave prognosis with predictably poor survival. On the other hand, those AIDS patients who initially develop only Kaposi's sarcoma in the absence of the infectious complications have a more favorable life expectancy [4, 12–14].

The early, usually asymptomatic and often faint lesions of AIDS-associated Kaposi's sarcoma (Figs. 1–8) can be easily overlooked by the patient and often misdiagnosed by the examining physician. Similar to classical Kaposi's sarcoma, the lesions of epidemic Kaposi's sarcoma can vary from flat macular patches to indurated papules and plaques or elevated nodules. The histopathology of the lesions at different stages is virtually identical for both the classical and epidemic varieties of Kaposi's sarcoma. In contrast to classical Kaposi's sarcoma in which a few,

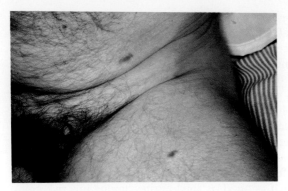

Fig. 1. Early red-patch-stage asymptomatic lesions of epidemic Kaposi's sarcoma. Note the ovoid shape. This 41-year-old, otherwise healthy homosexual male discovered these "spots" by chance. Of all AIDS-associated Kaposi's sarcoma's 95% are seen in homosexual men with AIDS

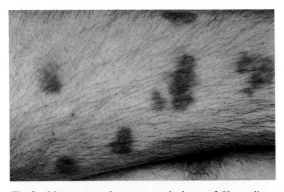

Fig. 2. Numerous plaque-stage lesions of Kaposi's sarcoma. These elongated, irregularly shaped, brown, similar elevated lesions were widespread over the skin of this 26-year-old homosexual male

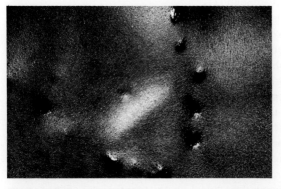

Fig. 3. Papular lesion of Kaposi's sarcoma seen in a black intravenous drug abuser. In dark-skinned individuals the lesions are hyperpigmented. Kaposi's sarcoma is not a common manifestation of AIDS in intravenous drug abusers with AIDS

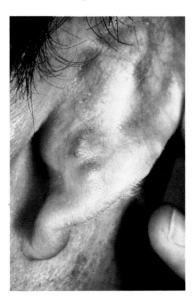

Fig. 4. Asymptomatic nodular lesion of Kaposi's sarcoma on the back of the ear in a homosexual man

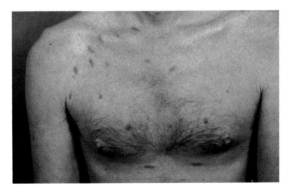

Fig. 5. Symmetrically distributed red-patch-stage lesions of Kaposi's sarcoma, widely disseminated in a 30-year-old bisexual man with AIDS. This bilateral, widespread lesion pattern is commonly seen in the epidemic form of Kaposi's sarcoma

localized, indolent tumors are commonly limited to the lower extremities, the lesions of Kaposi's sarcoma in the AIDS patient usually become numerous very quickly and are often widespread, showing a remarkable tendency to follow a unique symmetrical pattern of distribution along Langer's lines (skin cleavage lines), which has not been seen with the classical form of Kaposi's sarcoma. Unlike the classical disease in which the rounded tumors may persist for several years, gradually increasing in size and number, the typically more oval or fusiform lesions of AIDS-related Kaposi's sarcoma appear and continue to develop anywhere on the skin surface, oral mucosa, or within visceral organs. The tumors tend to increase in number and grow rapidly in size, with coalescence of neighboring lesions throughout the course of the disease. Patch-, plaque-, and nodular-stage lesions may be

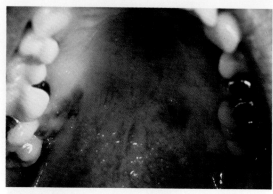

Fig. 6. Dark red, asymptomatic lesions of AIDS-related Kaposi's sarcoma found on the hard palate of a 23-year-old homosexual male who had no cutaneous lesions but had already experienced an episode of *P. carinii* pneumonia. He eventually developed multiple tumor lesions on his legs and trunk

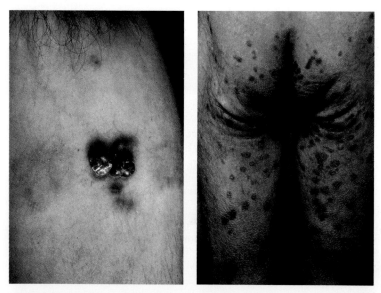

Fig. 7 *(left).* Nodular tumor lesions of Kaposi's sarcoma in a 47-year-old homosexual male of Italian extraction who had had the disease since 1980. His disease showed an indolent but slowly progressive course over 5 years (similar to that seen in classical Kaposi's sarcoma). He eventually died of multiple opportunistic infections. He was found to be seropositive for HIV antibodies

Fig. 8 *(right).* Advanced, widely disseminated epidemic Kaposi's sarcoma in a 36-year-old homosexual man who developed multiple opportunistic infections during the 2-year course of his disease

present simultaneously in the same anatomic locations in a patient with AIDS-related Kaposi's sarcoma.

The lesions of AIDS-related Kaposi's sarcoma may vary in color from pale pink through red or purple to bluish brown, and when the lesions are seen in dark-skinned individuals, they are hyperpigmented. The size of lesions can vary greatly in size, from 1–2 mm to several centimeters in diameter. The early flat, patch-stage lesions of epidemic Kaposi's sarcoma can be mistaken for other skin conditions, including traumatic bruises, melanomas, hemangiomas, or purpura. As the lesions evolve, they often become elevated and develop into thickened plaques. At this stage the lesions can resemble neoplasms associated with secondary syphilis, pityriasis rosea, lichen planus, sarcoidosis, insect bites, intradermal nevi, carcinomas, and cutaneous lymphomas, among others. Neighboring patch- and plaque-stage lesions may enlarge, coalesce, and develop into nodular tumors. Nodular lesions of Kaposi's sarcoma may resemble benign elevated nevi, neurofibromas, dermatofibromas, basal-cell carcinomas, or melanomas [15].

On occasion, patients with AIDS may be totally free of skin or mucosal lesions, with the first manifestations of Kaposi's sarcoma being detected by the discovery of foci of the tumor in the biopsies of enlarged lymph nodes or by the development of tumor lesions in visceral organs such as the lungs, gastrointestinal tract, spleen, liver, or kidneys [16–18]. Eventually, almost all of the AIDS patients with Kaposi's sarcoma develop mucocutaneous lesions during the course of their disease.

Clinically, Kaposi's sarcoma, especially as seen in the AIDS patient, appears to be a multicentric neoplasm in which each of the lesions arise de novo alone or in clusters at the same or distant sites. The multifocal distribution pattern with a predilection for the skin suggests that, with the exception of malignant melanoma, Kaposi's sarcoma does not behave like most other metastastic malignant tumors [19]. Among thousands of freshly dissociated tumor cells from tissue biopsies examined under the microscope very few cells in mitosis have been detected. Unlike the ease with which most malignant neoplasms can be grown in tissue culture, several in vitro attempts to grow, passage, and establish continuous cell lines of Kaposi's sarcoma tumor cells in tissue culture have been unsuccessful (personal observation, 1987).

Etiology of Kaposi's Sarcoma

The etiology of this fascinating, rare, and unusual neoplasm has remained a mystery since its first description over 100 years ago. In the case of AIDS-associated Kaposi's sarcoma, it has been hypothetically suggested that there may be one or more yet to be identified cofactors peculiar to the homosexual life-style which especially predisposes certain immunosuppressed homosexual males infected with HIV to develop this particular neoplasm. Even prior to the AIDS epidemic a number of potential contributory factors had been implicated to play a significant etiologic role in the evolution of this rare neoplasm. These include genetic predisposition, chemical or environmental factors, past or current infections with various bacteria or viral agents such as cytomegalovirus, the repression or expression of an oncogene, and the possible induction of tumor growth factors in an immunologically deficient host. The specific roles and interactions of one or more of these co-factors in the development of Kaposi's sarcoma, especially in the AIDS patient, are currently under investigation [20].

Treatment of AIDS-Related Kaposi's Sarcoma

The cause of death in patients with AIDS is almost always one or more of the severe opportunistic infections to which these patients are susceptible, and succumb. Although Kaposi's sarcoma is rarely the direct cause of death in patients with AIDS, there are clinical circumstances that warrant local or systemic treatment of the tumors of Kaposi's sarcoma in this patient population. Cosmetically disturbing red in purple tumor lesions, especially on the face or other exposed parts of the body, respond well to various local treatment modalities. The tumors of Kaposi's sarcoma are extremely sensitive to radiation therapy. Temporary palliative effects may also be achieved with local electrocauterization and curettage, surgical excision, and sometimes intralesional injections of chemotherapeutic agents such as vinblastine or bleomycin [4]. Cryotherapy with topical liquid nitrogen has been found to be useful in removing the small and more superficial tumor lesions with satisfactory cosmetic results (personal observations, 1987). Topical application of 1% dinitrochlorbenzene (DNCB) solution has been reported anecdotally to help resolve individual tumor lesions (personal observations, 1987). It should be noted that in some cases particular lesions of Kaposi's sarcoma have spontaneously disappeared without any form of treatment, even as new lesions have appeared at neighboring or distant sites in the same patient.

When rapidly progressive and disseminated mucocutaneous or systemic disease occurs, or when extensive systemic tumor involvement may compromise the functions of vital organs such as the lungs, systemic chemotherapy may be the physician's only recourse to provide temporary relief of disease progression. The administration of chemotherapeutic agents such as adriamycin, etoposide (VP16), bleomycin, or vinblastine have been successfully employed either as single agents or in combination, resulting in temporary reduction in the size of existing tumors, and may retard the continuous development of new lesions [4]. The decision to institute systemic chemotherapy to control Kaposi's sarcoma in AIDS patients should be considered with great caution since the risk of further compromising their already defective immune systems with these drugs is considerable and may render these individuals even more vulnerable to the dangers of infectious complications. Systemic administration of α-interferon has been shown to have a beneficial effect, causing at least temporary tumor regression in some AIDS patients with Kaposi's sarcoma [21–23]. Although the local and systemic therapy of AIDS-associated Kaposi's sarcoma may cause partial tumor regression and thereby provide transient palliation, none of these treatments has been shown significantly to influence the overall survival of these patients [4].

Treatment of Opportunistic Infections

The major medical efforts in AIDS patients, including those who develop Kaposi's sarcoma, at this time must concentrate on the accurate diagnosis of the various life-threatening opportunistic infections to which these patients are prone in order to provide the most specific and effective treatments available as soon as possible.

Antiretroviral Therapy

At this time, tremendous emphasis is being placed on development of drugs to control the insidious and progressive immunological deterioration and other biologic damage due to the underlying HIV infection in patients with AIDS. Recently, the first of a promising generation of antiretroviral agents, azidothymidine (AZT), a drug that inhibits the production of the enzyme reverse transcriptase, thereby interfering with HIV replication, has been shown to be therapeutically beneficial in a selected group of ARC and AIDS patients; it decreased mortality and the frequency of development of opportunistic infections, and appears at least to temporarily prolong life [24]. At present there are no effective immunomodulatory treatments available to reconstitute the AIDS patient's severely depleted immunological defense.

The major role of the physician caring for patients with AIDS at this time is in making an accurate and rapid diagnosis and instituting proper treatments for each of the multiple opportunistic infections experienced by these patients, which can not only reduce the morbidity and delay the inevitable mortality associated with this disease but also help to improve the quality of life of these unfortunate individuals during the brief course of their devastating illness.

References

1. Centers for Disease Control (1981) Pneumocystis pneumonia. MMWR 30: 250–252
2. Centers for Disease Control (1981) Follow-up on Kaposi's sarcoma and pneumocystis pneumonia. MMWR 30: 409
3. Friedman-Kien AE, Laubenstein L, Marmor M et al. (1981) Kaposi's sarcoma and pneumocystis pneumonia among homosexual men – New York and California. MMWR 30: 250–252
4. Krigel RL, Friedman-Kien AE (1985) Kaposi's sarcoma in AIDS. In: DeVita VT, Hellman S, Rosenberg SA (eds) AIDS: etiology, diagnosis, treatment and prevention. Lippincott, New York
5. Haverkos HW (1987) Factors associated with the pathogenesis of AIDS (1987) J Infect Dis 156: 251–257
6. Kaposi M (1872) Idiopathisches multiples Pigment-Sarkom der Haut. Arch Dermatol Syphil 4: 265–272
7. Safai B (1984) Kaposi's sarcoma: a review of the classical and endemic forms. Ann NY Acad Sci 437: 373–381
8. Templeton AC (1976) Kaposi's sarcoma. In: Andrade R, Gumport SL, Popkin GL, Rees (eds) Cancer of the skin, vol 2. Saunders, Philadelphia, pp 1183–1225
9. Harwood A, Osoba D, Hofstader M, Goldstein C et al (1979) Kaposi's sarcoma in recipients of renal transplants. Am J Med 67: 759–765

10. Haverkos HW (1981) Kaposi's sarcoma and nitrite inhalants. Adv Biochem Therap (in press)
11. Ziegler JL, Abrams DI (1985) In: DeVita VT, Hellman S, Rosenberg SA (eds) AIDS: etiology, diagnosis, treatment and prevention. Lippincott, Philadelphia, pp 223–233
12. Friedman-Kien AE, Laubenstein L, Rubinstein P et al. (1982) Disseminated Kaposi's sarcoma in homosexual men. Ann Intern Med 96(I): 693–700
13. Friedman-Kien AE, Greene J (1984) Aquired Immune Deficiency Syndrome. In: Petersdorf RG, Adams RD, Brouswald E, Isselbacher KJ, Marttin JB, Wilson JD (eds) Harrison's principles of internal medicine update, vol IV. Mc Graw Hill, New York (1986)
14. Navia BA, Jordan BD, Price RW (1986) The AIDS dementia complex: I. clinical features. Ann Neurol 19: 517–524
15. Friedman-Kien AE, Ostreicher R (1984) Overview of classical and epidemic Kaposi's sarcoma. In Friedman-Kien AE, Laubenstein LJ (eds) AIDS: the epidemic of Kaposi's sarcoma and opportunistic infections. Masson, New York, pp 23–34
16. Horowitz L, Stern JO, Segarra S (1984) Gastrointestinal manifestations of Kaposi's sarcoma and AIDS. In: Friedman-Kien AE, Laubenstein LJ (eds) AIDS: The epidemic of Kaposi's sarcoma and opportunistic infections. Masson, New York
17. Mildvan D, Mathur U, Enlow R et al. (1982) Persistent generalized lymphadenopathy among homosexual males. MMWR 31: 249–251
18. Metroka CE (1984) Generalized lymphadenopathy in homosexual men. In: Friedman-Kien AE, Laubenstein LJ (eds) AIDS: the epidemic of Kaposi's sarcoma and opportunistic infections. Masson, New York, pp 73–79
19. Giraldo G, Beth E, Coeur P et al. (1972) Kaposi's sarcoma: a new model in the search for viruses associated with human malignancies. J Natl Cancer Inst 49: 1495
20. Haverkos HW (1987) Factors associated with the pathogenesis of AIDS. J Infect Dis 156: 251–257
21. Krown SE, Real FX, Cunningham-Rundles S et al. (1983) Interferon in the treatment of Kaposi's sarcoma. Letter to the editor. N Engl J Med 309: 923
22. Groopman JE, Gottlieb MS, Goodman J et al. (1984) Recombinant alpha-2 interferon therapy for Kaposi's sarcoma associated with the aquired immune deficiency syndrome. Ann Intern Med 100: 671
23. Rios A, Mansell P, Dewell G et al. (1984) The use of lymphoblastoid interferon in the treatment of acquired immunodeficiency syndrome related Kaposi's sarcoma (abstract). Proc Am Soc Clin Oncol 3: 63
24. Fischl MA, Richman DD, Grieco MH et al. (1987) The efficacy of azidothymidine (AZT) in the treatment of patients with AIDS and AIDS-related complex. N Engl J Med 317: 185–191

Malignant Lymphomas in Patients with or at Risk for AIDS in Italy*

S. Monfardini**

Division of Medical Oncology, Centro di Riferimento Oncologico,
Via Pedemontana Occidentale, 33081 Aviano (Pordenone), Italy

Introduction

Besides Kaposi's sarcoma and other tumors such as the squamous carcinoma of the tongue and the cloacogenic carcinoma of the anorectum [2, 5, 6, 9, 10, 11, 12, 19, 21, 23, 24] malignant lymphomas have been shown to be one of the major problems among the neoplastic complications of the acquired immunodeficiency syndrome (AIDS) [1, 7, 14, 15, 17, 26, 29, 30]. According to North American experience, non-Hodgkin's lymphomas in patients with AIDS or with AIDS-related clinical conditions present at an advanced stage, concentrated in extranodal and often unusual locations, notably in the central nervous system (CNS). Disease confined to the lymph nodes is uncommon. These lymphomas are predominantly high-grade B-cell neoplasms classified as immunoblastic, lymphoblastic, and Burkitt-like lymphomas. A variety of severe opportunistic infections and Kaposi's sarcoma affects these patients. The association with AIDS is strengthened by the regular demonstration of reversed ratios of helper (T4$^+$) and suppressor (T8$^+$) lymphocytes in the peripheral blood and by the presence of antibodies to HIV [8]. The prognosis is dismal: response to chemotherapy does not positively affect median survival. Mortality rates analyzed according to histological grade are higher than the currently reported rates in other comparable patient populations [30].

Hodgkin's disease in patients at risk for or with AIDS also appears with unusual features compared to those of the general population developing this disease. The presentations described have been atypical with advanced stage, and response to therapy has been poor, with a very brief period of survival [1, 25, 26, 27].

* Partially supported by a grant of the Associazione Italiana per la Ricerca sul Cancro and by a grant of the Regione Friuli-Venezia Giulia.

**For the Italian Cooperative AIDS & Tumor Group (GICAT): U. Tirelli (Pordenone), E. Vaccher (Pordenone), G. Ambrosini (Trento), A. Andriani (Roma), R. Barbieri (Milano), I. Bianco Silvestroni (Roma), G. Broccia (Cagliari), T. Chisesi (Vicenza), G. Fassio (Bergamo), M. Gobbi (Bologna), F. M. Gritti (Bologna), G. Lambertenghi Deliliers (Milano), F. Lanza (Ferrara), A. Lazzarin (Milano), F. Lombardi (Milano), G. Luzi (Roma), C. Malleo (Palermo), F. Mandelli (Roma), G. Mariani (Roma), R. Maserati (Pavia), E. A. Parrinello (Verona), N. Piersantelli (Genova), R. Proto (Brindisi), F. Puppo (Genova), G. Rezza (Roma), A. M. Rosci (Roma), G. Rossi (Brescia), A. Sinicco (Torino), A. Tognetti (Pisa), F. Gavosto (Torino), R. Foà (Torino).

The majority of cases of malignant lymphomas in patients at risk for or with AIDS in the United States have been reported in homosexuals, thus leading to the conclusion that in this risk group malignant lymphomas are more common than in other high-risk patients such as intravenous drug abusers (IVDA) [8].

Presently in Europe little information is available on the neoplastic complications of AIDS, although medical oncologists and hematologists are aware from their personal experience or contacts with colleagues that such cases are beginning to be observed in Western Europe as well. So far only one article dealing with the pathological characteristics of malignant lymphomas in patients with AIDS has been published in France [22], and only sporadic cases have been reported in other countries of the European Community [3, 16, 20,]. Table 1 summarizes the available information on non-Hodgkin's lymphomas and Hodgkin's disease in persons with AIDS or at risk for AIDS in Europe.

In view of the scarcity of data (on only 24 patients in Europe), this report has been updated with some additional information quite recently provided by a single national group in Europe through the observation of more than 90 cases of malignant lymphomas in patients with AIDS or at risk for AIDS [18].

Table 1. Malignant lymphomas in persons with or at risk for AIDS in Europe

Authors	Number of patients	Risk group	Diagnosis of PGL/AIDS	Clinicopathological characteristics
Non-Hodgkin's lymphomas				
Lev et al. 1984 [16]	1	Homosexual	AIDS	High-grade NHL in association with Kaposi's sarcoma
Payan et al. 1984 [20]	1	Homosexual	AIDS	Primary CNS lymphoma (large-cell immunoblastic lymphoma)
Casadei and Gambacorta 1985 [3]	1	IVDA	AIDS	Primary CNS lymphoma with a simultaneous *Toxoplasma gondii* infection of the brain
Raphael et al. 1986 [22]	16	not stated	AIDS 100%	Immunoblastic cell lymphoma 69%, Burkitt's lymphoma 19% Extranodal sites 69% (CNS, bone marrow, mucocutaneous sites) PGL preexistent to NHL 50% Median survival 9 months
Hodgkin's disease				
Raphael et al. 1986 [22]	5	not stated	PGL 60%	PGL preexistent to HD 60%

PGL, persistent generalized lymphadenopathy; *IVDA*, intravenous drug abuser; *NHL*, non-Hodgkin's lymphoma; *CNS*, central nervous system.

Patients and Methods

At the Centro di Riferimento Oncologico of Aviano (Pordenone) and at the Clinica Medica I of the University of Turin, an Italian cooperative study group was organized in November 1986 with the aim of examining the incidence and outcome of malignant lymphomas in persons with AIDS or at high risk for AIDS in Italy.

A total of 1962 questionnaires were sent to members of the Italian Society for Medical Oncology, Hematology, and Immunology and to selected specialists on infectious diseases. These investigators were asked to identify all known patients at risk for AIDS (homosexuals, IVDA, hemophiliacs, the polytransfused) in whom a malignant lymphoma (non-Hodgkin's lymphoma or Hodgkin's disease) had developed between January 1980 and May 1987. By July 1987 268 completed questionnaires had been returned. A revised and integrated form was then sent to investigators (at 36 centers) who had previously reported cases of malignant lymphomas in order to better specify information regarding initial localizations, clinical stage, treatment response, toxicity, development of AIDS-associated conditions, and survival from time of treatment to death or to July 1987. The criteria used to diagnose persistent generalized lymphadenopathy (PGL) and AIDS conform to those established by the Centers for Disease Control [4]. Actuarial survival was determined by the method of Kaplan and Meyer [13].

Results

By July 1987, 71 cases of non-Hodgkin's lymphomas and 24 cases of Hodgkin's disease had been reported from the various centers in Italy. One patient was observed before 1983 and another before 1984, while the remaining cases have been observed at an increasing rate since 1984: five patients in 1984, 16 in 1985, 38 in 1986, and 19 in 1987. Not all data, including those on follow-up, were generally available in all cases, due to the peculiar features of this population of patients, such as the frequent change of address and of physician, imprisonment, and other economic and practical problems connected with intravenous drug abuse. Data on six registered cases are not yet available.

Table 2 shows the presently available information on persons in Italy at risk for AIDS with non-Hodgkin's lymphomas. (In each of the clinicopathological characteristics reported in this table as well as in the following, the denominator refers to the number of patients about whom information was available). The patients were predominantly male (85%). The majority of these patients with non-Hodgkin's lymphomas had AIDS, while only a small number presented PGL or the AIDS-related complex (ARC). One patient was only HIV-positive; three patients at risk (one polytransfused, one hemophiliac, and one IVDA) were HIV-negative. Overall, there was a prevalence of IVDA over homosexuals and polytransfused and hemophiliacs. In one HIV-positive patient no risk factor could be detected. Median age was 27 years. High-grade histology was present in 51/60 patients (85%), with a consistent percentage of these showing Burkitt-like histology (35%). Extranodal presentations at onset were clear in all but two patients (48/50) for whom information was available. Initial sites of disease were: CNS alone in 13 cases,

Table 2. Non-Hodgkin's lymphomas in persons with or at risk for AIDS in italy

Total number of patients: 71 (data available on 68)
Sex: 57/67 men (85%), 10/67 women (15%)
Median age: 27 years (range, 19–64)
HIV seropositivity 62/65 (95%)

Diagnosis

PGL	AIDS	ARC	Only HIV+
3/60 (4%)	59/68 (87%)	1/68 (1%)	1/62 (2%)

Risk Group

IVDA	Homo-sexual	IVDA-Homosexual	Poly-transfused	Hemo-philiac	"Not at risk"
46/66 (70%)	12/66 (18%)	5/66 (8%)	1/66 (2%)	1/66 (2%)	1/66 (2%)

Grade

Low	Intermediate	High	High, Burkitt-like
2/60 (3%)	7/60 (12%)	51/60 (85%)	11/31 (35%)

Stage

I	II	III	IV
14[a]/53 (26%)	2/53 (4%)	3/53 (6%)	34/53 (64%)

[a] 13/14 CNS, 1/14 lung
PGL, persistent generalized lymphadenopathy; *IVDA*, intravenous drug abuser; *ARC*, AIDS-related complex.

bone marrow in 14, liver in 17, spleen in 11, gastrointestinal tract in ten, skin in six, heart in three, lung in five, ovary in one, kidney in three, pancreas in two, adrenal gland in one, and larynx in one. In one case non-Hodgkin's lymphoma was associated with Kaposi's sarcoma, while in another case the diagnosis of angioimmunoblastic lymphadenopathy preceded the development of the lymphoma. Opportunistic infections at onset were present in 55% of evaluable patients (31/56).

Table 3 reports the presently available data on persons at risk for AIDS or with AIDS and Hodgkin's disease in Italy. As in the case of those with non-Hodgkin's lymphomas, these patients were predominantly male (90%). Almost half of the patients with Hodgkin's disease had PGL, only four had AIDS and two ARC. Four patients were only HIV-positive, and one patient at risk (IVDA) was HIV-negative. Again, the majority of patients were IVDA. Among the histological varieties, lymphocytic predominance was not represented. Of all patients, 70% had stage III or IV disease. Unusual initial extranodal presentation occurred in one patient with CNS involvement, while the other patients with stage IV disease had liver or bone marrow involvement. In this group the median age was also low (24 years). Opportunistic infections at onset were present in only one out of 17 patients (6%) who could be evaluated.

PGL was associated with non-Hodgkin's lymphomas in 68% of patients (27/40) and to Hodgkin's disease in 83% (15/80). PGL preceded the development of non-Hodgkin's lymphomas in 59% of cases (16/27) and in 92% of cases with Hodgkin's disease (11/12). In only two cases of non-Hodgkin's lymphoma with CNS

Table 3. Hodgkin's disease in persons with or at risk for AIDS in Italy

Total number of patients: 24 (data available on 21)
Sex: 19/21 men (90%), 2/21 women (10%)
Median age: 24 years (range 20–37)
HIV Seropositivity: 19/20 (95%)

Diagnosis

PGL	AIDS	ARC	Only HIV+
9/13 (47%)	4/19 (21%)	2/19 (11%)	4/19 (21%)

Risk Group

IVDA	Homosexual	IVDA + Homosexual
18/21 (86%)	0	3/21 (14%)

Histology

LP	NS	MC	LD
0	7/17 (41%)	8/17 (47%)	2/17 (12%)

Stage

I	II	III	IV
1/17 (6%)	4/17 (24%)	6/17 (35%)	6/17 (35%)

PGL, persistent generalized lymphadenopathy; *IVDA,* intravenous drug abusers; *ARC,* AIDS-related complex; *LP,* lymphocytic predominance; *NS,* nodular sclerosis; *MC,* mixed cellularity; *LD,* lymphoid depletion.

involvement did PGL precede the lymphoma. The median latency between PGL and non-Hodgkin's lymphomas was 12 months and only 8 months for PGL and Hodgkin's disease.

Almost half (47%) of patients with non-Hodgkin's lymphomas for whom information on therapy was available (22/47) could not receive any antineoplastic therapy due to rapid disease progression, treatment refusal, or death (postmortem diagnosis). Twenty patients received various combination chemotherapy regimens (CVP, CHOP, ProMACE-MOPP, ProMACE/CYTABOM, and others), three patients received combination chemotherapy and radiotherapy, but only five patients achieved complete and ten partial remission. The four cases of complete remission for which information is available lasted 17, 22, 25, and 33 months.

At the time of the present report 46 patients have died. As regards the cause of death, progression of the disease accounted for 41% of cases (19/46), opportunistic infections for 26% (12/46), both for 2% (1/46), and bone marrow toxicity, coagulation intravascular disease, and heart failure for 2% each (1/46). In 11 patients the cause of death could not be ascertained. The median survival period of patients with non-Hodgkin's lymphomas was only 5 months (see Fig. 1).

Out of 21 patients with Hodgkin's disease 18 could be evaluated as regards therapy. These were treated with mustine, oncovin, procarbazine, and prednisone (MOPP) alternated with adriamycin, bleomycin, vinblastine, and dacarbazine (ABVD) (eight patients), MOPP followed by ABVD (four patients), MOPP alone (four patients) and ABVD alone (two patients). Complete remission was observed in 5/18 patients, while 6/18 patients achieved a partial remission. Information on the duration of complete remission is available in only 3/5 patients: response lasted 2, 10, and 37 months. The median survival of patients with Hodgkin's disease

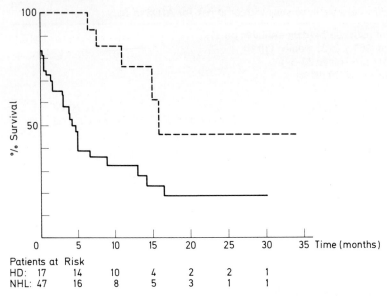

Fig. 1. Survival rate for AIDS patients with non-Hodgkin's lymphomas (*NHL, solid line;* $n=47$) and those with Hodgkin's disease (*HD, broken line;* n = 17); $\chi_1^2 = 9.39$, $p = 0.002$. Diagnoses of malignant lymphoma was made postmortem in 11 patients with non-Hodgkin's lymphoma and in one with Hodgkin's disease

was 16 months (Fig. 1). Four died of opportunistic infection and two of coagulation intravascular disease.

With regard to the evolution in the four patients at risk for AIDS but HIV-negative, the only patient with Hodgkin's disease at the time of this report is alive and in complete remission after 2 years from initial diagnosis, while two patients with high-grade non-Hodgkin's lymphoma presented as rapid progression of the disease as other patients who were HIV positive. No proper information is presently available on the course of the disease of the one remaining HIV-negative patient with non-Hodgkin's lymphoma.

Discussion

Non-Hodgkin's lymphoma of Burkitt's type was one of the earliest recognized manifestations of AIDS [30]. Non-Hodgkin's lymphomas of high-grade histology or of CNS origin which occur in seropositive patients are diagnostic of AIDS, according to the Centers for Disease Control (CDC) definition [4], also in absence of opportunistic infections or Kaposi's sarcoma. Three large series of AIDS-related non-Hodgkin's lymphomas [1, 15, 30] and two of Hodgkin's disease [25, 27] have been reported from the United States. Both non-Hodgkin's lymphomas and, to a lesser extent, Hodgkin's disease in the North American experience present extra-nodal involvement and are related to a short survival. Recently, the pathological characteristics of 21 cases associated with AIDS have been described in Paris, while so far only sporadic cases have been reported in the rest of Europe [3, 16, 20, 22].

This article suffers the obvious limitation of a retrospective cooperative study on a problem whose importance has been emerging only recently – but not necessarily at the time when the clinical observations could be made. However, this study is the result of the only nationwide inquiry conducted in Europe.

These preliminary data reveal for the first time the presence in Italy of a consistent number of malignant lymphomas among persons at high risk for AIDS. This information confirms that patients with non-Hodgkin's lymphomas have an increased incidence of high-grade subtypes, particularly of the Burkitt type, that they present advanced stage disease with frequent extranodal involvement, and that they have a short median period of survival. The majority of cases with non-Hodgkin's lymphomas has been observed in IVDAs.

As regards Hodgkin's disease, the incidence of advanced stages (III and IV) and of extranodal localizations was rather high in comparison to the average population of patients with Hodgkin's disease without AIDS or not at risk for AIDS, but unusual localizations were rare (only one case with CNS involvement). As in the instance of non-Hodgkin's lymphomas, the Italian cases of Hodgkin's disease were predominantly among IVDAs and not homosexuals. Also, in Italian patients the occurrence of Hodgkin's disease was correlated with a shorter survival time.

This survey confirms that, in contrast to what has been observed in the general population of this age group, non-Hodgkin's lymphomas seem to be more common than Hodgkin's disease in persons at high risk for or with AIDS in Italy. The fact that in this series the majority of cases could be observed beginning only in 1983 is in keeping with the general tendency of a 2-year delay in the spread of the epidemic in Europe compared with the United States.

In the majority of patients with PGL was associated with and preceded the development of malignant lymphoma. In fact, some patients presenting PGL were referred to some of the oncological centers participating in this cooperative study because of the clinical diagnosis of lymphoma. Initial clinical presentations of PGL are similar to those of malignant lymphoma, often being accompanied by malaise, fever, night sweats, weight loss, and splenomegaly [28]. The potential diagnosis of malignant lymphoma should therefore be considered in a patient with PGL. Biopsy at more than one site may be necessary in the investigation of these patients. As time elapses and clinical conditions bring the clinical suspicion of a lymphoma, repeated biopsy may be required.

Contrary to the North American experience, it has been shown that, at least in Italy, malignant lymphomas are more frequent in IVDA than in homosexuals. An increased risk for Hodgkin's disease and non-Hodgkin's lymphomas in the New York area among prisoners (of whom more than 40% have a history of drug abuse) has, in fact, already been presented, but the problem has not yet been described in full probably because of the difficulty in studying patients with such a concentrated burden of human vicissitudes: drug abuse, jail, AIDS, and lymphoma.

The problem of AIDS-related tumors deserves attention not only from a clinical point of view but also in consideration of the possible progress achievable in understanding the etiology and pathogenesis of the neoplastic complications of

AIDS. This report shows that a relatively large set of case material is presently available in Europe, allowing for a better study of the virological, immunological, pathological, and clinical aspects of the problem. The need for a careful collection of data on European patients at risk for AIDS with malignant lymphomas and also for other tumors should then receive priority attention. Along this line, the results of the work of this Italian cooperative study group on AIDS and related tumors may possibly be considered as the first step to a better focus on the present situation in Europe.

References

1. Ahmed T, Worsher G, Stahl R, et al. (1985) Increased risk for Hodgkin's disease (HD) and non-Hodgkin's lymphomas (NHL) in a population at risk for AIDS. Proc Annu Meet Am Soc Clin Oncol 4: 5
2. Biggar RJ, Horm J, Lubin JH, et al. (1985) Cancer trends in a population at risk of acquired immunodeficiency syndrome. JNCI 4: 793-794
3. Casadei GP, Gambacorta M (1985) A clinico-pathological study of seven cases of primary high-grade malignant non-Hodgkin's lymphoma of the central nervous system. Tumori 71: 501-507
4. MMWR (1985) Case definition of AIDS revised. MMWR 34: 373-375
5. Centers for disease control task force on Kaposi's sarcoma and opportunistic infections (1982) Report. Epidemiologic aspects of the current outbreak of Kaposi's sarcoma and opportunistic infections. N Engl J Med 306: 248-252
6. Cooper MS, Patchefsky AS, Marks G (1979) Cloacogenic carcinoma of the anorectum in homosexual men: an observation of four cases. Dis Colon Rectum 22: 557
7. Diffuse undifferentiated non-Hodgkin's lymphoma among homosexual males in the United States (1982) MMWR: 277-279
8. Editorial (1986) Malignant lymphomas in homosexuals. Lancet 1: 193-194
9. Friedman-Kien AE, Laubenstein LJ, Raubenstein P, et al. (1982) Disseminated Kaposi's sarcoma in homosexual men. Ann Intern Med 69: 693-697
10. Gottlieb GJ, Ragaz A, Vogel JV, et al. (1981) A preliminary communication on exclusively disseminated Kaposi's sarcoma in young homosexual men. Am J Dermatopathol 3: 111-114
11. Gottlieb GJ, Ackerman B (1982) Kaposi's sarcoma: an extensively disseminated form in young homosexual men. Hum Pathol 13: 882-892
12. Hymes KB, Greene JB, Marcus A, et al. (1981) Kaposi's sarcoma in homosexual men – a report of eight cases. Lancet 2: 598-600
13. Kaplan EL, Meier P (1958) Nonparametric estimation from incomplete observations. J Am Stat Assoc 53: 457-481
14. Jaffe ES, Clark J, Steis R, et al. (1985) Lymph node pathology of HTLV-associated neoplasms. Cancer Res 45: 4662S-4664S
15. Joachim HL, Cooper MC, Hellmann GG (1985) Lymphomas in men at high risk of acquired immunodeficiency syndrome (AIDS). Cancer 51: 2831-2842
16. Lev HJ, Schneider J, Hardmeier T, et al. (1984) Kaposi's sarcoma and malignant lymphoma in AIDS. Virchows Arch 403: 205-212
17. Levine AM, Gill PS, Burkes RL, et al. (1985) Retrovirus and malignant lymphoma in homosexual men. JAMA 14: 1921-1925
18. Monfardini S, Tirelli U, Vaccher E, et al. (1987) Malignant lymphomas in patients with or at risk for AIDS in Italy. In: Third international conference on malignant lymphoma, Lugano, p 49 (abstract 58)
19. Myskowski PL, Romano JF, Safai B (1983) Kaposi's sarcoma in young homosexual men. Cutis 29: 31-34

20. Payan MJ, Gambarelli D, Routy JP, et al. (1984) Primary lymphnode of the brain associated with AIDS. Acta Neuropathol (Berl) 64: 7880
21. Peters RK, Mack TM (1983) Patterns of anal carcinoma by gender and marital status in Los Angeles County. Br J Cancer 48: 629
22. Raphael M, Tulliez M, Bellefqih S, et al. (1986) Les lymphomes et le SIDA. Ann Pathol 6: 278-281
23. Safai B, Koziner B (1985) Malignant neoplasms in AIDS. In: De Vita Jr VJ, Hellmann S, Rosenberg SA (eds) AIDS – etiology, diagnosis, treatment and prevention. Lippincott, Philadelphia, pp 213-222
24. Safai B (1985) Kaposi's sarcoma and other neoplasms in acquired immunodeficiency syndrome. In: Gallin JI, Fauci AS (eds) Advances in host defense mechanisms. Raven, New York, pp 59-73
25. Schoeppel SL, Hoppe RT, Dorfman RF, et al. (1985) Hodgkin's disease in homosexual men with generalized lymphadenopathy. Ann Intern Med 102: 68-70
26. Schoeppel S, Hoppe R, Abrams D, et al. (1986) Hodgkin's disease (HD) in homosexual men: the San Francisco Bay area experience. Proc Annu Meet Am Soc Clin Oncol 5: 3
27. Unger PD, Strauchen JA (1986) Hodgkin's disease in AIDS complex patients. Report of four cases and tissue immunologic marker studies. Cancer 58: 821-825
28. Vaccher E, Tirelli U, Zagonel V, et al. (1987) Clinical and laboratory findings in persistent generalized lymphadenopathy (PGL) versus malignant lymphoma (ML). In: International symposium on immunobiology in clinical oncology and immune dysfunctions, Nice, p 117 (abstract 191)
29. Ziegler JL, Miner RC, Ronsenbaum E, et al. (1982) Outbreak of Burkitt's lymphoma in homosexual men. Lancet 2: 631-633
30. Ziegler JL, Beckstead AJ, Volberding PA, et al. (1984) Non-Hodgkin's lymphoma in 90 homosexual men. N Engl J Med 311: 565-570

HIV-Related Hematological Neoplasias in France*

J.-M. Andrieu, M. Toledano, M. Raphael, J.-M. Tourani, and
B. Desablens**

Laennec Hospital, 42 Rue de Sévres, 75007 Paris, France

Introduction

In 1981 the unexpected appeareance of opportunistic infections and Kaposi's sarcoma in homosexual men in the United States marked the beginning of the AIDS epidemic [8]. Shortly thereafter the observation of an increasing number of male homosexual subjects suffering from high-grade non-Hodgkin's lymphomas [6, 15, 16] resulted in the inclusion of this hematological malignancy in the Centers for Disease Control (CDC) definition of AIDS [4]. As early as 1983 the retrovirus responsible for this major immunodeficiency state, now called human immunodeficiency virus (HIV), was discovered [3, 11]. Since then the HIV infection epidemic has been spreading rapidly by means of sexual and intravenous transmission routes in America as well as in Africa and Europe. The discovery of different types of hematological and non hematological malignancies in AIDS patients and HIV-positive subjects led us to create a French register of HIV-related neoplasia. This paper reports the first 68 cases of hematological malignancies identified in this register between 1983 and June 1987.

Patients and Methods

An HIV-related neoplasia register was opened in January 1987. Included in this register were all tumors, except Kaposi's sarcoma, occurring in HIV-seropositive subjects with or without AIDS. We proceeded in the following manner: hematologists, oncologists, radiation therapists, specialists of infectious diseases, and pathologists at 25 French university hospitals were contacted by telephone and asked whether they were aware of the presence of HIV-seropositive patients suffering or having suffered from a malignant tumor. If the answer was positive and the contacted physician agreed to participate in the register, a questionnaire was sent to him. This questionnaire concerned the following points:

1. Demographic characteristics of the patient: age, sex, ethnic group, country of origin.
2. Date of the first positive results of serological tests (ELISA or Western blot).

* This work was supported by Ligue Nationale contre le cancer and AREMAS.
**For the French Registry of HIV-Associated Tumors.

3. Type of contamination: male homosexuality, heterosexual contact, drug-abusers' syringe sharing, blood transfusion, etc.
4. Date of discovery of the tumor and characteristics of the tumor: histological type and dissemination stage.
5. Clinical status of HIV infection just before or at the time of discovering the tumor, evaluated according to our Laennec system of stages [1]. This system allows classification of HIV-seropositive subjects without AIDS into three clinical classes: (a) absence of symptoms (apparently healthy carriers); (b) presence of persistent generalized lymphadenopathies; (c) presence of constitutional symptoms – fever, night sweats, diarrhea, weight loss – or oral thrush. AIDS patients, forming a fourth group, were subclassified into those with opportunistic infections, Kaposi's sarcoma, and severe neurological disorders.
6. Biological status of HIV infection, as evaluated by blood count, T4 and T8 subsets, and globulin electrophoresis.
7. Type of treatment – surgery, radiation therapy, and/or chemotherapy – and its efficiency and toxicity.
8. Date of the last clinic visit or date of death, with tumor status as well as clinical and biological condition of HIV disease at that time. The cause of death was also recorded.

Once the completed questionnaire was received by the organizing committee, it was studied in detail. In the event of insufficient data, a resident was sent to the hospital in question in order to study the medical files and to discuss the case with the physician. Afterwards data were stored in a computer and analyzed by means of a specific evaluative program.

Results

As of June 1987 clinical data on 68 patients were available for analysis. These came from 14 participating institutions.

Table 1 shows the type and number of hematological neoplasia retrospectively recorded each year. Of all cases 74% were non-Hodgkin's lymphomas (NHL), and 22% were Hodgkin's disease (HD). The remaining 4% included one case of acute

Table 1. Types and number of HIV-related hematological neoplasias retrospectively recorded each year

Types of HIV-related hematological neoplasia	Years of diagnosis					1983–1987[a]
	1983	1984	1985	1986	1987[a]	
Non-Hodgkin's lymphomas	3	6	15	18	8	50
Hodgkin's disease	–	1	6	4	4	15
Acute lymphoblastic leukemia	–	–	1	–	–	1
Acute myeloblastic leukemia	–	–	1	–	–	1
Waldenström's macroglobulinemia	–	–	–	–	1	1
All hematological neoplasias	3	7	23	22	13	68

[a] Until June 1987.

lymphoblastic leukemia, one of acute myeloblastic leukemia, and one of Waldenström's macroglobulinemia.

Table 2 summarizes the demographic characteristics of the patients and gives the patterns of HIV transmission: 95% of the patients with NHL and 100% of those with HD were men. In NHL the intravenous route of contamination represents 15% of cases (plus 5% of patients infected by both sexual and intraveinous routes) whereas it represents 50% of the cases in HD ($P<0.05$, using the χ^2 test).

Table 3 summarizes the characteristics of the 50 cases of NHL. High-grade histology ws recorded in 34 of these (68%) and intermediate- and low-grade in 14 (28%) and in two cases respectively. Most NHL cases were at advanced stages (40 at stages III or IV, six with extranodal sites without nodal disease).

Clinical status of the underlying HIV disease could be evaluated in 42 cases. Thirteen patients (31%) already suffered from AIDS (eight instances of NHL diag-

Table 2. Demographic characteristics and types of HIV contamination of 68 HIV-related hemological malignancies

	Non-Hodgkin's lymphomas ($n=50$)	Hodgkin's disease ($n=15$)	Other malignancies ($n=3$)
Age (years)			
Range	22–66	24–42	26–39
Median	39	31	27
Sex			
Male	45	15	3
Female	5	–	–
Area of origin			
Europe	35	12	2
North Africa	2	–	1
Central Africa	2	–	–
West Africa	1	–	–
South America	2	1	–
Carribean	2	–	–
Asia	1	–	–
No information	5	2	–
Type of HIV contamination			
Males			
Homosexuality	29	6	1
Heterosexuality	6[a]	1	–
Syringe sharing	4[b]	7	2
Blood transfusion	2	–	–
Females			
Heterosexuality	2	–	–
Syringe sharing	1	–	–
Blood transfusion	2	–	–
No information	4	1	–

[a] Includes four cases in Africa.
[b] Includes two cases of syringe sharing and homosexuality.

Table 3. Characteristics of 50 HIV-related cases of non-Hodgkin's lymphomas

Histology (working formulation)	n
High grade	
Burkitt's type	16
Large-cell immunoblastic	17
lymphoblastic	1
Intermediate grade	
Diffuse large cell	13
Diffuse mixed	1
Low grade	
Small lymphocytic plasmocytoid	1
Follicular mixed	1
Clinical stages (Ann Arbor)	n
Extranodal only	
Central nervous system	4
Psoas	1
Anorectal	1
Nodal (+ extranodal)	
Stages I + II	4
Stages III + IV	40
Clinical status of underlying HIV disease	n
HIV seropositive without AIDS	
No symptoms	14
Persistent generalized lymphadenopathies	5
Constitutional symptoms or oral thrush	10
AIDS	
Opportunistic infections	11[a]
Opportunistic infections and Kaposi's sarcoma	1
Kaposi's sarcoma	1
No information	8

[a] Includes eight cases of lymphoma diagnosed at autopsy.

nosed at autopsy). On the other hand, 29 instances of NHL occurred in HIV-seropositive subjects without AIDS. Of these, 14 were completely asymptomatic ("healthy" carriers).

Various types of treatments were given. Of the 31 patients for whom treatment information was available, 21 had received multiagent chemotherapy (mostly cyclophosphamide, hydroxydaunorubicin, oncovin, prednisolone CHOP – combination), eight had received chemotherapy plus irradiation (with bone marrow rescue in two cases), and irradiation alone was given in two cases. In these 31 patients the initial complete remission rate reached 53% (16/31). Twenty-nine patients died within the 24 months following the diagnosis of NHL (a further eight were diagnosed at autopsy). The cause of death was lymphoma progression in 18 cases, opportunistic infections in seven, and treatment-related non opportunistic infections in five. The overall 24-month actuarial survival rate was 12% (Fig. 1), with an actuarial median survival of 5 months. There was no difference in the survival rate ac-

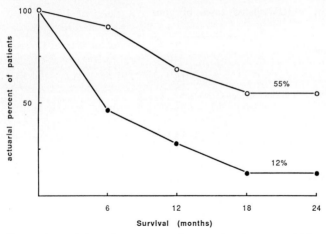

Fig. 1. Actuarial survival curves of HIV-related non-Hodgkin's lymphomas *(solid circles)* and Hodgkin's disease *(open circles)*. Deaths among those with non-Hodgkin's lymphomas, 29/42; among those with Hodgkin's disease, 5/15

Table 4. Characteristics of 15 HIV-related cases of Hodgkin's disease

	n
Histology (Lukes-Collins)	n
Lymphocytic predominance (I)	1
Nodular sclerosis (II)	5
Mixed cellularity (III)	7
Lymphoid depletion (IV)	1
Unclassified	1
Clinical stages (Ann Arbor)	n
I	2
II	3
III	4
IV	6
Clinical status of underlying HIV disease	n
HIV seropositive without AIDS	
No symptoms	4
Persistant generalized lymphadenopathies	3
Constitutional symptoms or oral thrush	4
AIDS	
Opportunistic infections	2
Kaposi's sarcoma	1
No information	1

cording to the histology or the clinical stage of the NHL. On the other hand, the clinical status of the underlying HIV infection did seem to play a role: the 24-month survival rate of the patients with no symptoms or with persistent generalized lymphadenopathies was 17% while it was only 8% in patients with constitutional symptoms or with AIDS ($p=0.056$, using the log-rank test).

Table 4 summarizes the overall characteristics of the 15 cases of HIV-related HD. Histological types II and III and advanced clinical stages (III and IV) were observed in 12/15 and 10/15 patients, respectively. The clinical status of the underlying HIV infection was recorded in 14/15 cases. Three patients already had AIDS when HD was diagnosed, and 11 were seropositive without AIDS; of these, four were completely asymptomatic before acquiring HD. Information concerning treatment was obtained in six cases: three had received multiagent chemotherapy – mustine, oncovin, procarbazine, prednisone (MOPP) and/or adriamycin, bleomycin, vinblastine, dacarbazine (ABVD) – and the had others focal or hemitorso irradiation. All six entered in complete remission. The overall 24-month actuarial survival rate of the 15 patients was 55% (Fig. 1). As of June 1987 five patients had died, four with opportunistic infection and one with evolutive HD.

Discussion

This paper reports the first 68 cases of hematological malignancies retrospectively recorded between 1983 and June 1987 in 14 university hospitals affiliated with the French HIV-related tumor register. We have previously documented this aspect of HIV infection in European cases [13]. Information concerning epidemiological features, histology, and extent of the tumor is of good quality, as is that on the clinical status of the underlying HIV infection and on the date of last follow-up. On the other hand, however, information concerning treatment of the tumor, its efficiency and toxicity, as well as immunological data concerning HIV infection are very scarce and inadequate, and these clearly need to be improved in the future. This study confirms, with a large number of cases of NHL, well-known features, such as high-grade histological types, presentation at advanced stages, increased extranodal and primary brain involvement, and bad prognosis despite an initially good response to chemotherapy. The underlying HIV infection seems to be the determinant for prognosis. Patients at early stages of HIV infection (without symptoms or with persistent generalized lymphadenopathies) who have a mean T4 cell count most frequently of over 400/ml have a better survival rate than do patients with advanced stages (constitutional symptoms and AIDS) who have a very low T4 cell count (generally under 100/ml). This had already been suspected by Ziegler [16] who identified different clinical outcomes among 66 HIV-related NHL patients according to prodromal manifestations. This no doubt explains the failure of such usual prognostic factors as histological subtypes and clinical stage [5].

Our 15 cases of HD occurring in HIV-infected subjects have the same histological and clinical patterns (prevalence of mixed-cell histology and of clinical stages III and IV) as already shown in other small series [2, 12, 14].

Interestingly, the route of HIV contamination in our group of subjects suffering from HD is intravenous in 50% of cases, whereas the corresponding rate in HIV-related NHL as well as in a large cohort of HIV-infected subjects (Laennec cohort) is only 15% ($p < 0.001$). Moreover, HD is not one of the malignancies observed with an incresed incidence after organ transplatation [7, 10]. This observation raises the question of an etiological agent of HD whose transmission by infected blood would be more efficient than by sexual routes; such an agent has been recently suspected as a retroviral particle [9].

This retrospective study, conducted through a questionnaire survey of 14 institutions, demonstrates the need for a large multicentric prospective study of HIV-related tumors in order to acquire a better understanding of the etiology and pathophysiology of NHL and HD and to design specific treatment strategies taking into account the immune defect of the underlying HIV infection. For this reason we are now engaged in the development of a national register of HIV-related tumors.

Acknowledgements. Participating institutions were the following: Ambroise Paré Hospital (Paris), Angers Hospital (Angers), Avicenne Hospital (Paris), Cimiez Hospital (Nice), Cochin Hospital (Paris), Gustave Roussy Hospital (Villejuif), Henri Mondor Hospital (Creteil), Hôtel Dieu Hospital (Paris), Laennec Hospital (Paris), Pasteur Institute Hospital (Paris), Paul Brousse Hospital (Villejuif), Pitie Salpetriere Hospital (Paris), Southern Hospital (Amiens), and Tenon Hospital (Paris). Participating physicians were the following: M. F. Auclerc, P. Casassus, A. Delmer, P. Dujardin, B. Dupont, M. Gentilini, P. Godeau, A. Goguel, E. Goldschmidt, J. Guerre, L. Guillevin, D. Machover, J.-P. Marie, C. Mayaud, B. Rio, W. Rozenbaum, D. Schaffo, D. Sicard, C. Theodore, M. Tulliez, and J. M. Ziza.

References

1. Andrieu JM, Even P, Venet A (1986) AIDS and related syndromes as a viral induced autoimmune disease of the immune system: an anti-MHC II disorder. Therapeutic implications. AIDS Res 3: 163–174
2. Baer DM, Anderson ET (1986) Acquired immune deficiency syndrome in homosexual men with Hodgkin's disease. Am J Med 80: 738–740
3. Barré-Sinoussi F, Chermann JC, Rey F et al. (1983) Isolation of a T-lymphotropic retrovirus from a patient at risk for acquired immune deficiency syndrome (AIDS). Science 220: 868
4. Centers for disease control (1985) Revision of the case definition of acquired immunodeficiency syndrome for national reporting - United States. Ann Intern Med 103: 402–403
5. Di Carlo EF, Ambrson JB, Metroka CE, Ballard P, Moore SA, Mouradian JA (1986) Malignant lymphomas and the acquired immunodeficiency syndrome. Arch Pathol Lab Med 110: 1012–1016
6. Doll DC, List AF (1982) Burkitt's lymphoma in a homosexual. Lancet 1: 1026–1027
7. Doyle TJ, Ventachalam KK, Maeda K, Saedd SM, Tilchen EJ (1983) Hodgkin's disease in renal transplant recipients. Cancer 51: 245–247
8. Gottlieb MS, Schroff R, Schauker HM, Weisman JD, Peng TF, Wolf RA, Saxon A (1981) Pneumocystis carinii pneumonia and mucosal candidiasis in previsusly healthy homosexual men: evidence of a new acquired immunodeficiency. N Eng J Med 305: 1425
9. Lesser J, Dormont D, Tourani JM, Schwartz O, Fleury H, Neveux Y, Audroin C, Andrieu JM (1987) Particules d'aspect retroviral et activité transcriptase inverse dans des cultures cellulaires dérivées de biopsies ganglionnaires de maladie de Hodgkin. CR Acad Sci (Paris) 305: 295–300
10. Penn I (1983) Lymphomas complicating organ transplantation. Transplant Proc 15: 2790–2797

11. Popovic M, Sarngadharam MG, Read E, Gallo RC (1984) Detection, isolation and continuous production of cytopathic retro-viruses (HTLV III) from patients with AIDS and pre-AIDS. Science 224: 497
12. Prior H, Goldberg AF, Conjalka MS, Chapman WE, Tay S, Ames ED (1986) Hodgkin's disease in homosexual men in AIDS-related phenomenon? Am J Med 81: 1085–1088
13. Raphael M, Tulliez M, Bellefqin S, Louvel A, Ziza JM, Rozenbaum W (1986) Les lymphomes et le SIDA. Ann Pathol 278: 281–286
14. Unger PD, Strauchen JA (1986) Hodgkin's disease in AIDS complex patients. Cancer 58: 821–825
15. Ziegler JL, Miner CR, Rosenbaum E, Lennette ET, Shillitoe E, Casavour C, Diew WL, Mintz L, Gershow J, Greenspan J, Beckstread J, Yamamoto K (1982) Outbreak of Burkitt's like lymphoma in homosexual men. Lancet 2: 631–633
16. Ziegler JL et al. (1984) Non-Hodgkin's lymphoma in 90 homosexual men. N Engl J Med 311: 565–569

Malignant Lymphomas in Patients with Human Immunodeficiency Virus Infection

E. M. Hersh and T. P. Miller

Section of Hematology and Oncology, Department of Internal Medicine,
University of Arizona Health Science Center, Tucson, AZ 85724, USA

Malignant lymphoma, particularly high-grade non-Hodgkin's lymphoma, has been shown to occur with increased incidence in a number of congenital immunodeficiency diseases, in autoimmune and inflammatory diseases, as well as in association with certain therapies [20]. The common denominator seems to be chronic immune stimulation associated with immunodeficiency or chemical immunosuppression. Table 1 lists the diseases and conditions showing this association. In ataxia telangiectasia an additional complicating factor is impaired DNA repair. Among the acquired immunodeficiency diseases several inflammatory conditions, including Sjögren's syndrome and Hashimoto's thyroiditis, combine an inflammatory and autoimmune disease with concurrent cellular immunodeficiency. The major new condition in this category of predisposing diseases is, of course, HIV infection. An incresed incidence of malignant lymphoma has also been seen in patients receiving immunosuppressive therapy. Chronic daily therapy with corticosteroids, azathioprine, alkylating agents, cyclosporin A, or combinations of these to maintain organ grafts or to suppress autoimmune and inflammatory diseases including rheumatoid arthritis and systemic lupus erythematosus, are all associated with an increase of 30 to several hundred times in the incidence of malignant lymphomas compared to that seen in the general population.

Table 1. Association of malignant lymphoma with other diseases and conditions

Disease-associated
  Congenital immunodeficiency diseases
    Ataxia telangiectasia
    Common variable immunodeficiency
    Wiskott-Aldrich syndrome
    Severe combined immunodeficiency disease
  Acquired immunodeficiency inflammatory diseases
    Sjögren's syndrome
    Hashimoto's thyroiditis
    Immunoblastic lymphadenopathy
    HIV infection
Immunosuppressive therapy associated
    Transplant recipients
    Autoimmune and inflammatory diseases
    Cancer chemotherapy/radiotherapy

The pattern of malignancy, particularly that of non-Hodgkin's lmyphoma is strikingly different in the various categories of disease associated with this increased incidence of malignancy [21]. Table 2 shows the relative frequency of non-Hodgkin's lymphoma and the other malignancies among organ transplant recipients, patients with autoimmune and inflammatory disease on immunosuppressive therapy, patients receiving cancer chemotherapy, those with congenital immunodeficiency, and those with AIDS. Non-Hodgkin's lymphoma is the dominant form of malignancy in individuals with organ transplants, immunosuppressive therapy, and congenital immunodeficiency diseases, accounting for 30%–60% of the cases of cancer with increased incidence. In AIDS, the predominant form of malignancy is Kaposi's sarcoma; non-Hodgkin's lymphoma accounts for less than 20% of the cases of malignancy. Clearly, cofactors play a role in this differential incidence; these may include age, type of immunosuppression, type of concurrent carcinogenic therapy, factors related to bone marrow proliferation (such as would be seen in patients receiving repeated courses of cancer chemotherapy), and concurrent infections such as with cytomegalovirus (CMV), Epstein-Barr virus (EBV), and herpes simplex virus (HSV).

Table 3 lists the AIDS-related malignancies which have been described thus far. Kaposi's sarcoma is the dominant form of malignancy, followed by malignant

Table 2. Malignancies showing increased frequency in association with immunodeficiency/immunosuppression

Organ transplants	Immuno-suppressive therapy	Cancer chemotherapy	Congenital immuno-deficiency	AIDS
NHL	NHL	Acute leukemia	NHL	KS
Skin/lips	Leukemia	NHL	Stomach	NHL
Cervix	Bladder	Bladder	Acute leukemia	Oral SSC
KS	KS	Common cancers	HD	Rectal SSC
Perineum				Skin
Vulva				HD

In each group the malignancies are listed in decreasing frequency from top to bottom. Skin and lip cancer is 60% squamous cell, 30% basal cell, and 10% melanoma.
NHL, non-Hodgkin's lymphoma; *KS,* Kaposi's sarcoma; *SSC,* squamous cell carcinoma; *HD,* Hodgkin's disease.

Table 3. AIDS-related malignancy

Kaposi's sarcoma
Malignant lymphoma
Oral squamous cell carcinoma
Anorectal carcinoma
Multiple myeloma solitary plasmacytoma
Prolymphocytic leukemia
Testicular carcinoma
Multiple primaries of the above

lymphoma [23]. There is also an incresed incidence of squamous cell carcinoma of the mouth, tongue, and pharynx. Anorectal squamous cell carcinoma and cloacogenic carcinoma were seen with increased incidence among homosexual men prior to the onset of the AIDS epidemic. Whether these have further increased since the onset of the epidemic is not entirely clear. Other malignancies which have been reported include multiple myeloma and solitary plasmacytoma, prolymphocytic leukemia, and testicular carcinoma. Whether these are truly of increased incidence is as yet undetermined. Finally, it is common to find patients who manifest two or even three of the above malignancies at the same time (usually Kaposi's sarcoma and malignant lymphoma) [11, 18].

Table 4 compares some features of non-Hodgkin's lymphoma among patients with AIDS to those in the general population [3, 4, 5, 14]. All non-Hodgkin's lymphoma in AIDS patients is of B-cell origin. Almost all cases are high-grade and are either small noncleaved or B-cell immunoblastic types, whereas in non-Hodgkin's lymphoma in the general population the most common histologies are follicular small cleaved-cell (low-grade) and diffuse large-cell lymphoma (intermediate-grade). The second striking clinical feature of AIDS-related lymphoma is the high incidence of unusual, limited extranodal disease at presentation, particularly involving the brain, anus and rectum, head and neck, lung, and liver as primary sites. This occurs in 20% of AIDS-related lymphomas as opposed to 1% or less in the general population. The third distinguishing feature of AIDS-related lympho-

Table 4. Comparison of malignant lymphoma in AIDS and in the general population

Parameter	AIDS	General population
Etiology[a]	Immunosuppression	Unknown
Cell of origin	B	B, T
Cell types	Small noncleaved (50%)	Follicular small cleaved (23%)
	B-cell immunoblastic (40%)	Diffuse large Cell (20%)
Grade	High	Various
Polyclonality	Common	Rare
EBV genome	Often present	Rare
c-*myc* translocated[b]	Yes	Yes
c-*myc* rearranged and/or truncated	Yes	No
Limited extranodal disease at presentation	20%	1%
Remission rate	High	High
Remission duration and survival	Short	Long
Hodgkin's disease		
Stage IV at presentation	80%	10%
Mixed-cellularity histology	85%	30

EBV, Epstein-Barr virus.
[a] Refers to non-Hodgkin lymphoma.
[b] In Burkitt-like lymphoma.

ma is the presence of B symptoms in 85% of cases compared to only 15% of cases in the general population. In Burkitt-like lymphomas the c-*myc* oncogene has been shown to be translocated as in the sporadic Burkitt-like lymphoma in the general population, but the gene is also rearranged, truncated, and associated with immunoglobulin secretion not generally observed in the sporadic cases [7, 12, 19]. The EBV genome is found in the majority of non-Hodgkin's lymphomas associated with HIV infection.

There are several reports of patients with HIV infection who also manifest Hodgkin's disease [22, 27]. Controversy exists as to whether the incidence is increased in HIV infection since the age distribution of HIV infection and Hodgkin's disease overlap. However, the stage at presentation (stages III and IV in 80% of Hodgkin's disease patients with HIV infection versus 10% in Hodgkin's disease patients in the general population) and the mixed-cellularity histologic type (in 85% of Hodgkin's disease patients with HIV infection versus 30% of cases in the general population) at least suggests that AIDS changes both the presenation and rate of progression of this disorder.

Given the above background, the following hypothesis can be generated (Fig. 1). HIV infection can directly induce polyclonal B-cell activation and can also stimulate macrophages which in turn induce T cells to produce growth factors such as B-cell growth factor (BCGF) and B-cell stimulating factor (BSF-1). HIV infection also induces T helper cell depletion and T-cell immunodeficiency. Polyclonal B-cell activation and this T-cell immunodeficiency result in augmentation of EBV infection of B cells and incresed proliferation of cells containing the EBV genome. This results in translocation and rearrangement of the c-*myc* oncogene. This in turn results in c-*myc* activation, oligoclonal B-cell proliferation, and ultimately monoclonal malignant transformation. At these steps, T-cell immunodeficiency will play a further permissive role. This results in malignant cells with the characteristics shown in Table 5. The cells have a monoclonal light-chain surface phenotype. Cytogenetic analysis shows an (8:14) translocation. Further analysis shows

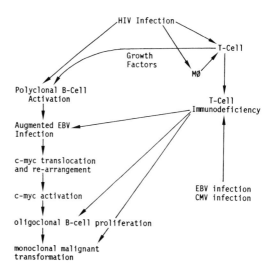

Fig. 1. Pathogenesis of Burkitt-like B-cell lymphoma in HIV infection. *EBV,* Epstein-Barr virus; *CMV,* cytomegalovirus; *M0,* macrophage

Table 5. Characteristics of malignant cells of HIV-infection-associated lymphoma

Surface phenotype	Monoclonal light chain
Genotype	(8:4) translocation
Immunoglobulin genes	Rearrangements, deletions
c-*myc* genes	Rearrangements
EBV genome	Expressed
HIV genome	Not present
T-cell antigen genes	Germline

EBV, Epstein-Barr virus.

immunoglobulin gene rearrangement, c-*myc* oncogene rearrangement, expression of the EBV genome, and absence of the HIV genome. The T-cell antigen genes have the germline configuration.

The first problem in the clinical management of AIDS-related lymphoma is diagnosis. Controversy has arisen as to whether patients with persistent generalized lymphadenopathy (PGL) [1] should undergo lymph node biopsy. In some series, lymph node biopsies have been almost uniformly negative in terms of revealing anything more than AIDS-associated follicular hyperplasia, while in others 10%–15% of biopsies have revealed other pathological conditions, such as Kaposi's sarcoma, malignant lymphoma, [6, 15]. *Mycobacterium avium* or *M. intracellulare* infection, and histoplasmosis since most patients with non-Hodgkin's lymphoma and Hodgkin's disease present with stage III or IV disease, we are obviously missing the diagnosis when the disease is in its early stages. Currently, our recommendations for lymph node biopsy in patients with HIV-associated lymphadenopathy are as follows: patients with atypical nodal presentations such as asymmetrical or hard lymph nodes, patients presenting with the B symptoms of fever, night sweats, and weight loss, or patients with prognostic factors as described by Abrams for progression of PGL to AIDS [1] should undergo biopsy. Repeated biopsy of suspicious nodal areas may be required.

As already noted, over 80% of patients with AIDS-related non-Hodgkin's lymphoma and Hodgkin's disease present with B symptoms and with stage III and IV disease. As described by DiCarlo and coworkers [4] the presenting sites in decreasing order of frequency include: lymph nodes, brain and meninges, bone marrow, gastrointestinal (GI) tract, head and neck area, skin, lung, and liver.

The responses to therapy with aggressive combination chemotherapy (CHOP, M-BACOD, etc.) and survival of patients with HIV infection associated malignant lymphomas are poor [4]. While almost 70% of patients achieve complete (CR) or partial remission (PR) (excluding patients with primary brain presentations) less than 30% show CR, and the median survival period is only approximately 5 months. This is due to recurrence and progression of lymphoma, but also to fatal opportunistic infection, dementia, etc.

Several unique extranodal presentations are worthy of special mention. Approximately 10% of AIDS-associated lymphomas present as primary brain disease [25, 26]. On computed tomography scans [13] these are usually single or multiple discrete lesions and less frequently bilateral low-density lesions, cerebral atrophy, or only equivocal findings. Most commonly, the patients present with confusion, lethargy, memory loss, hemiparesis, or aphasia. Less commonly, seizures, cranial nerve palsies, or headache may be the presenting manifestations. There are a number of intercurrent problems in the diagnosis and management of CNS lymphoma worthy of mention. One must distinguish cerebral toxoplasmosis, meningeal infections, other cerebral infections, and cerebral Kaposi's sarcoma from malignant lymphoma. In addition, these conditions may occur concomitantly with brain lymphoma. HIV-associated cerebral atrophy, which can manifest the same symptoms as malignant lymphoma, must be distinguished and may also occur concomitantly, as may progressive multifocal leukoencephalopathy. Finally, as in the management of systemic lymphoma, intercurrent systemic opportunistic infections can complicate and interfere with the management of the primary brain lymphoma. Standard treatment for brain lymphoma after biopsy confirmation, is radiotherapy. However, the response to treatment is usually only transient and incomplete, and patients often die within a few months. New approaches should be explored.

Another extranodal presentation of interest is anorectal lymphoma [2]. Alone and in combination with nodal disease this is seen in 10% of AIDS patients with lymphoma compared to less than 1% of lymphomas in the general populations. It is usually high-grade, it is not (as in the general population) usually associated with primary GI lymphoma at other sites. It also has a poor prognosis. Again, localized radiotherapy is the management approach most frequently used. However, initial systemic chemotherapy designed for cure might be more effective and might avoid the problem of dissemination of disease during treatment of the local area [17].

A recent development possibly portends a new problem of AIDS-associated lymphoma/leukemia in the future. Serological evidence of HTLV-I and HTLV-II infection has been found in the intravenous drug abuser risk group. Thus, Guroff et al. [24] found that of 56 intravenous drug abusers 9% were infected with HTLV-I, 18% with HTLV-II, 41% with HIV, and 18% with HTLV-I or -II plus HIV. This can only be expeced to increase. It is conceivable that not only will such patients have increased susceptibility to non-Hodgkin's lymphoma and Hodgkin's disease but will also become susceptible to the malignancies associated with HTLV-I and -II, namely T-cell leukemia/lymphoma and hairy-cell leukemia.

Clearly, new approaches are needed for effective therapy of HIV infection related malignant lymphomas. Efforts must be made to improve and develop early diagnosis. It is possible that careful peripheral blood lymphocyte phenotyping and repeated lymph node biopsies with phenotyping may provide one avenue to securing an earlier diagnosis. Our suggestions for the study of improvement in therapy are given in Table 6. Strategies may be developed to combine antiretroviral drugs with conventional antitumor chemotherapy, perhaps in an intermittent or cyclic fashion. Since CMV infection plays a very important role in the progression of AIDS, it may be possible to intersperse therapy with anti-CMV drugs such as DHPG. Because of the myelosuppressive and immunosuppressive effects of standard combination chemotherapy, the use of colony-stimulating factors (CSF) such as granulocyte macrophage CSF (GM-CSF) between courses of chemotherapy may improve chemotherapy tolerance and the CR rate. Alternatively, we may consider other antitumor therapeutic approaches. Monoclonal antibodies directed

Table 6. New approaches needed for effective therapy of HIV infection-related malignant lymphoma

Additions to conventional chemotherapy
  Antiretroviral drugs (azidothymidine)
  Anti-CMV drugs (dehydroxyphenylglycol)
  Colony-stimulating factors granulocyte macrophage CSF)
Other therapeutic approaches
  Monoclonal antibodies
  Interferons and other cytokines
T-cell immunorestoration
  Diethyldithiocarbamate
  Thymic hormones
  Interleukin 4
Reduction of c-*myc* product
  Plicamycin
  Anti-sense RNA

against the surface phenotype of malignant cells, including the antiidiotype approach pioneered by Meeker and coworkers [16] may provide antitumor activity without immunosuppression. Similarly, the use of interferons [8] or other cytotoxic cytokines, when combined with conventional modalities, could conceivably control the lymphoma, again while either themselves having antiretroviral effects or at least not further compromising host defense mechanisms. Interferon alone would not be expected to have major activity in these high-grade lymphomas. Another approach which should be considered would be to use concomitant immunorestorative therapy. There is already preliminary evidence that thymic hormones [10] and synthetic immunorestoratives such as diethyldithiocarbamate [9] can improve the symptomatology, reduce the lymphadenopathy, and improve the T-cell function of patients with AIDS and the AIDS-related complex (ARC). It would be relatively easy to conduct investigations comparing conventional chemotherapy to conventional chemotherapy plus these immunorestoratives. Finally, it has been proposed that reduction of the c-*myc* product by plicamycin or the use of anti-sense RNA to its messenger RNA might also result in control of this disease category.

Since few, if any, centers have enough patients to investigate these avenues alone, we propose that an international study group for the diagnosis and treatment of AIDS-related lymphomas is established, and that protocols are set up to investigate these and other modalities to be added to or substituted for conventional therapy. Without such an approach, it is unlikely that further progress will be made in either better understanding or managing malignant lymphoma as a complication of HIV infection.

References

1. Abrams DI (1986) Lymphadenopathy related to the acquired immunodeficiency syndrome in homosexual men. Med Clin N Am 70: 693–706
2. Burkes RL, Meyer PR, Gill PS, Parker JW, Rasheed S, Levine AM (1986) Rectal lymphoma in homosexual men. Arch Intern Med 146: 913–915
3. Caccamo D, Pervez NK, Marchevsky A (1986) Primary lymphoma of the liver in the acquired immunodeficiency syndrome. Arch Pathol Lab Med 110: 553–555
4. DiCarlo EF, Amberson JB, Metroka CE, Ballard P, Moore A, Mouradian JA (1986) Malignant lymphomas and the acquired immunodeficiency syndrome. Arch Pathol Lab Med 110: 1012–1016
5. Duncan ED, Miller HJ, McKeever WP (1986) Non-Hodgkin's lymphoma, HTLV-III/LAV, and HTLV-III/LAV antibody in the wife of a man with transfusion-acquired AIDS. Am J Med 81: 898–900
6. Farthing CF, Henry K, Shanson DC, Taube M, Lawrence AG, Harcourt-Webster JN, Gazzard B (1986) Clinical investigations of lymphadenopathy, including lymph node biopsies, in 24 homosexual men with antibodies to the human T-cell lymphotropic virus type III (HTLV-III). Br J Surg 73: 180–182
7. Groopman JE, Sullivan JL, Mulder C, Ginsburg D, Orkin SH, O'Hara CJ, Falchuk K, Wong-Staal F, Gallo RC (1986) Pathogenesis of B-cell lymphoma in a patient with AIDS. Blood 67: 612–615
8. Gutterman JU, Blumenshein GR, Alexanian R et al. (1986) Leukocyte interferon induced tumor regression in human breast cancer, multiple myeloma and malignant lymphoma. Am Intern Med 93: 399–406
9. Hersh EM, Petersen E, Yocum DE, Gorman RS, Darragh JM (1986) Dose response study of diethyldithiocarbamate (DTC or imuthiol) in patients (pts) with ARC and AIDS. Proc Am Soc Clin Oncol 6: 2
10. Hong R (1986) Reconstitution of T-Cell deficiency by thymic hormone or thymus transplantation therapy. Clin Immunol Immunopathol 40: 136–141
11. Katner H, Pankey GA, Flaum MA, Dalovisio JR, Cortez LM, DeShazo RD (1986) Kaposi's sarcoma with a non-Hodgkin's lymphoma: its association in male homosexual with human T-cell lymphotropic virus type III infection. Arch Intern Med 146: 393–394
12. Lanfrancone L, Pelicci P-G, Dalla-Favera R (1986) Structure and expression of translocated c-myc oncogenes: specific differences in endemic, sporatic and AID-associated forms of Burkitt lymphomas. Curr Top Microbiol Immunol 132: 257–265
13. Lee YY, Bruner JM, Tassel PV, Libshitz HI (1986) Primary central nervous system lymphoma: CT and pathologic correlation. AJR 147: 747–752
14. Levine AM, Gill PS (1987) AIDS-related malignant lymphoma: clinical presentation and treatment approaches. Oncology 1: 41–45
15. Levine AM, Meyer PR, Gill PS, Burkes RL, Krallo M, Aguilar S, Parker JW (1986) Results of initial lymph node biopsy in homosexual men with generalized lymphadenopathy. J Clin Oncol 4: 165–169
16. Meeker TC, Lowder J, Maloney DG et al. (1985) A clinical trial of anti-idiotype therapy for B-cell malignancy. Blood 65: 1349–1363
17. Miller TP, Jones SE (1983) Initial chemotherapy for clinically localized lymphomas of unfavorable histology. Blood 62: 413–418
18. Mitsuyasu RT, Colman MF, Sun NCJ (1986) Simultaneous occurence of Hodgkin's disease and Kaposi's sarcoma in a patient with the acquired immune deficiency syndrome. Am J Med 80: 954–958
19. Pellicci P-G, Knowles DMII, Arlin ZA, Wieczorek R, Luciw P, Dina D, Basilico C, Dalla-Favera R (1986) Multiple monoclonal B-cell expansions and c-myc oncogene rearrangements in acquired immune deficiency syndrome – related lymphoproliferative disorders: implications for lymphomagenesis. J Exp Med 164: 2049–2060

20. Penn I (1986a) Cancer is a complication of severe immunosuppression. Surg Gynecol Obstet 162: 603–610
21. Penn I (1986b) The occurrence of malignant tumors in immunosuppressed states. Prog Allergy 37: 259–300
22. Prior E, Goldberg AF, Conjaika MS, Chapman WE, Tay S, Ames ED (1986) Hodgkin's disease in homosexual men an AIDS-related phenomenon? Am J Med 81: 1085–1088
23. Purtilo DT, Linder J, Volsky D (1986) Acquired immune deficiency syndrome (AIDS). Clin Lab Med 6: 3–26
24. Robert-Guroff M, Weiss SH, Giron JA, Jennings AM, Ginzburg HM, Margolis IB, Blattner WA, Gallo RC (1986) Prevalence of antibodies to HTLV-I, -II, and -III in intravenous drug abusers from an AIDS endemic region. JAMA 255: 3133–3137
25. Rosenberg NL, Hochberg FH, Miller G, Kleinschmidt-DeMasters BK (1986) Primary central nervous system lymphoma related to Epstein-Barr virus in a patient with acquired immune deficiency syndrome. Ann Neurol 20: 90–102
26. So YT, Beckstead JH, Davis RL (1986) Primary central nervous system lymphoma in acquired immune deficiency syndrome: a clinical and pathological study. Ann Neurol 20: 566–572
27. Unger PD, Strauchen JA (1986) Hodgkin's disease in AIDS complex patients: report of four cases and tissue immunologic marker studies. Cancer 58: 821–825
28. Ziegler JL (1987) The article reviewed. Oncology 1: 46

Malignant Lymphomas and HIV Infection

D. Huhn and M. Serke

Klinikum Charlottenburg, Freie Universität Berlin,
Spandauer Damm 130, 1000 Berlin, FRG

According to the literature, malignant lymphomas occur in 5%–20% of patients infected with HIV [1–10]. Malignant lymphoma was shown in one study to be the immediate cause of death, as determined at autopsy, in 2% of 110 patients with AIDS [11], whilst Kaposi's sarcoma was the cause of death in 5% of patients. In the following, results published by various authors will be discussed, in addition to results relating to 16 of our own patients.

Findings in more than 200 cases of malignant lymphoma in HIV-infected patients have been published so far [1–10], including those relating to our 16 patients (Table 1). In instances in which immunological marker investigations were conducted, all patients were found to have lymphomas of the B-cell type. In 85% of cases lymphoma of high- or intermediate-grade malignancy was detected, in 8% lymphoma of low malignancy, and in 5% Hodgkin's disease.

Most patients showed advanced-stage lymphoma and organ involvement. The pattern of organ involvement in 161 HIV-positive patients was compared to that

Table 1. Malignant lymphoma in HIV-infected patients, as reported from other centers [2–10] and in our own patients [1]

Number of patients	Non-Hodgkin's lymphoma			Hodgkin's disease	Reference
	High and intermediate malignancy	Low malignancy	Questionable		
27	21	6			2
14	13		1		3
21	17	1		3	4
16	12	3		1	1
1		1			5
90	82	6	2		6
1				1	7
1				1	8
4				4	9
29	29				10
204 (100%)	174 (85%)	17 (8%)	3 (2%)	10 (5%)	

Table 2. Organ involvement by malignant lymphoma in 161 HIV-infected patients [1–9] compared with patients in the Kiel Lymphoma Study Group (1975–1980) [12]

Patient group	Number of patients	Organ Involvement			
		Central Nervous System	Gastro-intestinal tract	Skin	Lungs
HIV patients	161	26%	21%	11%	7%
Kiel study					
IB	83	3%	19%	8%	0
CB	157	6%	20%	6%	0
LB	60	7%	15%	10%	0

IB, immunoblastic lymphoma; *CB*, centroblastic lymphoma; *LB*, lymphoblastic lymphoma (including 11 patients with Burkitt-type lymphoma).

of 300 patients with lymphoma of high-grade malignancy, who were studied by the Kiel Lymphoma Study Group in a multicenter trial (Table 2). CNS involvement was more frequent in HIV-infected patients (26%) than in patients who were probably HIV-negative (5%–6%). Involvement of the gastrointestinal tract was found in about 20% of cases in both groups, but it was more extensive and multilocular in HIV-infected patients. Involvement of the skin occurred with a frequency of about 10% in both groups; involvement of the lungs was observed in HIV-positive patients (7%), but never in patients of the Kiel Lymphoma Study Group.

Results of malignant lymphoma treatment in HIV-positive patients as well as their prognosis depend mainly on the stage of the immunodeficiency disorder [6]. The mortality and morbidity rates for 66 HIV-positive patients with malignant lymphoma treated by cytostatics are (at the time of writing) as follows:

1. Twelve men were asymptomatic when malignant lymphoma was diagnosed: four have died, one is alive but ill, and seven are living and without evidence of lymphoma.
2. Thirty-three men had generalized lymphadenopathy before the diagnosis of lymphoma: 19 have died, seven are alive but ill, and seven are alive and well.
3. Twenty-one men had AIDS before the diagnosis of lymphoma: 15 have died, four are alive but ill, and only two are well.

Of the 66 patients mentioned above 38 have died: half from progressive lymphoma and half from opportunistic infections.

Results in Our Own Patients

The mean age of our 16 patients was 39 years (range, 22–63). The age of patients with lymphoma of low malignancy did not differ from that in those with lymphoma of high malignancy. There was one 28-year-old patient with plasmocytoma. Immunohistochemical investigation on frozen or paraffin-embedded material was performed with 11 patients. B-cell lymphoma was detected in all but two patients; in patient number 4 (see Table 3) results were open to question, and T-cell lymphoma was under discussion. In patient number 6 all immunological markers were negative, including myeloic ones. Cytochemistry revealed focal activity of acid phosphatase, but no activity of peroxidase and no PAS-positive material. The diagnosis, therefore, was acute undifferentiated leukemia.

Four patients showed stages 3 S or 3 E (Table 4), the remaining 12 patients showed stage 4. Bone marrow was involved in four cases and the liver in five. In three patients lymphoma manifestations of the gastrointestinal tract were detected; in each of these cases the involvement was multilocular and extensive. Six patients suffered from lymphoma of the central nervous system; this was of intracerebral location in four, and lymphoma-induced meningeosis was detected in two (numbers 6 and 14).

The T4/T8 ratio was below 0.5 in nine patients (Table 5). IgG in the serum was elevated in four and was low in one. IgA was elevated in five and IgM in two patients.

The lymphoma was treated in six patients (Table 6). Complete remission was achieved in three cases by cytostatics and in one by involved field irradiation. In one patient (number 14) with leukemic manifestation of centroblastic lymphoma a remission of lymph node involvement was obtained; the patient died some months later from progressive disease of the central nervous system. One patient

Table 3. Age, diagnosis, and immunohistochemical markers in 16 patients with HIV infection and malignant lymphoma

Patient number	Age[a]	Diagnosis	Immunological markers
1	46	Plasmocytoma	κ,
2	28	Plasmocytoma	λ, HLA-DR
3	34	Centrocytic	B cell
4	34	Lymphoblastic	T cell (?)
5	34	Lymphoblastic	n.d.
6	49	Lymphoblastic	all neg., AUL
7	43	Large B cell	B cell, κ
8	50	Large B cell	lymphocyte, Ki1
9	36	Large B cell	n.d.
10	58	Large B cell	B cell, κ
11	43	Large B cell	n.d.
12	63	Immunoblastic	B cell, λ
13	41	Immunoblastic	n.d.
14	27	Centroblastic	B cell, κ, μ
15	22	Burkitt-type	CALLA, κ, HLA-DR
16	24	Hodgkin's, MC	n.d.

[a] Mean 39.5 years.
κ, λ, kappa and lambda light chains of immunoglobulin, μ, heavy chains; *AUL*, acute undifferentiated leukemia; *HLA-DR*, human leukocyte antigen DR; *CALLA*, common leukemia antigen; *Ki1*, activation antigen detected by Ki1 antibody; *MC*, mixed cellularity-type of Hodgkin's disease, n.d., no data.

Table 4. Stage and organ involvement in 16 patients with HIV infection and malignant lymphoma

Patient number	Stage	Organ involvement
1	3 S	–
2	4	BM, kidney
3	3 E	Abdominal wall
4	4	GI
5	4	Liver
6	4	BM, CNS
7	4	GI, CNS, liver
8	4	BM, liver
9	3 S	–
10	4	Liver
11	4	CNS
12	4	CNS
13	4	GI, CNS
14	4	BM, CNS
15	4	Liver
16	3 S	–

BM, bone marrow; *GI,* gastrointestinal tract; *CNS,* central nervous system.

Table 5. T4/T8 ratio and serum immunoglobulins in 15 patients with HIV infection and malignant non-Hodgkin's lymphoma

Patient number	T4/T8	IgG	IgA	IgM
1	0.8	2585 ↑	178	390 ↑
2	0.3	–	–	–
3	–	–	–	–
4	0.35	1941 ↑	457 ↑	210
5	0.3	640 ↓	200	200
6	2.3	–	–	–
7	0.3	1590	554 ↑	263
8	0.5	1470	628 ↑	176
9	–	950	496 ↑	67 ↓
10	0.2	–	–	–
11	0.2	1850	547 ↑	134
12	0.02	2242 ↑	398	115
13	0.2	2340 ↑	350	392 ↑
14	0.05	732	162	114
15	1.0	1240	187	102

↑, elevated; ↓, below normal.

Table 6. Treatment of six patients with HIV infection and malignant lymphoma

Patient number	Treatment	Result
3	COP-BLAM, IF-$\frac{1}{2}$	CR
4	CHOP	CR
6	ADM, VCR, Pred., Aspar. MTXit, $\frac{1}{2}$ CNS	CR
14	COP-BLAM, MTXit	PR
15	CHOP	PD
16	IF-$\frac{1}{2}$	CR

PD, progressive disease; *CR*, complete remission; *PR*, partial remission; *COP-BLAM*, cyclophosphamide, vincristine, prednisolone, bleomycin, methotrexate; *IF-$\frac{1}{2}$*, involved field irradiation; *CHOP*, cyclophosphamide, vincristine, adriamycin, prednisolone; *Aspar.*, asparaginase; *MTXit*, methotrexate given intrathecally; *ADM*, adriamycin; *VCR*, vincristine; *Pred.*, prednisolone.

(number 15) suffered from extensive involvement of the gastrointestinal tract and lymph nodes and died from progressive lymphoma.

Conclusions

In keeping with the results from other centers, we found a prevalence of malignant lymphoma of high malignancy and of B-cell type. Classification according to the nomenclature of the Kiel study is often difficult and equivocal. There is no characteristic histological or immunohistochemical type of malignant lymphoma in HIV-infected patients, but many different subtypes were observed, and each case was unique in terms of its histological or immunological pattern.

In contrast to the findings with non-HIV-infected patients, malignant lymphomas of low malignancy may be seen in rather young patients, the involvement of the central nervous system is frequent, and involvement of the gastrointestinal tract may be very extensive and severe.

AIDS-related lymphadenopathy is not a prerequisite for the later development of malignant lymphoma, and in two of our patients primary involvement of the central nervous system was detected at autopsy (patient numbers 11 and 12).

Treatment with cytostatics was well tolerated by three of our patients, resulting in complete remission. In one of these patients the last cycles of chemotherapy included the additional administrations of azidothymidine without unusual problems of cytopenia. In one patient (number 6) severe thrombocytopenia improved 3 days after the start of treatment with cytostatics and prednisolone, pointing to an immunological mechanism of thrombocytopenia.

The etiology of malignant lymphoma in HIV-infected patients remains open to discussion. Epstein-Barr virus genomes could be not detected in the lymphoma cells of one patient tested (Dr. Wolff, Munich). The impairment of T helper cells and especially of the dendritic reticular cells of the lymph follicles will have to be considered.

References

1. Serke M, Huhn D, Dienemann D, Eichenlaub D, Serke S (1988) HIV-related malignant lymphomas - a clinical and pathological study of 13 cases. Klin Wochenschr (in press)
2. Gill S, Lavine AM, PR et al. (1985) Primary central nervous system lymphoma in homosexual men. Clinical, immunological, and pathologic features. Am J Med 78: 742-748
3. Kalter SP, Riggs SA, Cabanillas F et al. (1985) Agressive Non-Hodgkin's lymphomas in immunocompromised homosexual males. Blood 66: 655-659
4. Ioachim HL, Cooper MC, Hellmann GC (1985) Lymphomas in men at high risk for acquired immune deficiency syndrome (AIDS). Cancer 56: 2831-2842
5. Zoller WG, Rübe Ch, Permanetter W, Hehlmann R, Goebel FD, Hübner G (1986) Erworbenes Immundefektsyndrom mit Thrombozytopenie, polymorphzelligem Immunozytom und Kryptosporidiose. AIDS-Forschung 1: 203-210
6. Ziegler JL, Beckstaed, JA, Volberding PA et al. (1984) Non-Hodgkin's lymphoma in 90 homosexual men. N Engl J Med 311: 565-570
7. Scheib RG, Siegel RS (1985) Atypical Hodgkin's disease and the acquired immunodeficiency syndrome. Ann Intern Med 102: 554
8. Robert NJ and Schneiderman H (1984) Hodgkin's disease and the acquired immunodeficiency syndrome. Ann Intern Med 100: 142
9. Schoeppel L, Hoppe RT, Dorfmann RF et al. (1985) Hodgkin's disease in homosexual men with generalized lymphadenopathy. Ann Intern Med 102: 68-70
10. DiCarlo EF, Amberson JB, Metroka CE et al. (1986) Malignant lymphomas and the acquired immunodeficiency syndrome. Arch Pathol Lab Med 110: 1012-1016
11. Vincent T, DeVita MD Jr, Discussants, Samuel Broder MD, Fauci AS, Kovacs MD, JA, Chabner BA MD (1987) Developmental therapeutics and the acquired immunodeficiency syndrome. Ann Intern Med 106: 568
12. Brittinger G, Bartels H, Common H et al. (1984) Clinical and prognostic relevance of the Kiel classification of Non-Hodgkin-lymphomas; results of a prospective multicenter study by the Kiel lymphoma study group. Hematol Oncol 2: 269-306

AIDS-Related Neoplasias in Switzerland

L. Schmid

Abteilung für Onkologie und Hämatologie, Medizinische Klinik C,
Kantonsspital, 9007 St. Gallen, Switzerland

Immunodeficiency and Cancer

It is generally agreed that the malignant tumours of individuals with HIV infections are in some way associated with a virus-induced T cell immunodeficiency. There is convincing epidemiological evidence that this is true for Kaposi's sarcoma and for non-Hodgkin's lymphoma (NHL).

In this context, however, one must be aware of the fact that in recent years a number of other examples for the immunogenesis of malignant tumours have been described. There are some rare congenital and acquired immunodeficiency syndromes which clearly show an increased incidence of malignant tumours. For example, about 12% of patients with ataxia telangiectasia and about 15% of those with Wiskott-Aldrich syndrome develop NHL (see table 1) [1, 2]. Interestingly, especially NHL of the B-cell type with an immunoblastic morphology is diagnosed in these patients. A high percentage of these instances of NHL show some sort of central nervous system involvement.

Patients treated with both chemo- and radiotherapy for Hodgkin's lymphoma have a statistically higher risk for development of NHL as well as for development of acute non-lymphatic leukaemias (Table 2) [3, 4]. The pathogenesis of these "secondary" tumours has been only partly elucidated. Immunodeficiency seems at least to some extent to play a role.

Renal transplant recipients who require long-term immunosuppressive therapy are also at risk for the development of malignant tumours (Table 2) [5]. The spectrum of tumour types is similar to that observed in individuals with HIV infections. A relatively high proportion of skin tumours (including Kaposi's sarcoma)

Table 1. Ataxia telangiectasia, Wiskott-Aldrich syndrome and cancer

Disorder	Type of tumour	Incidence	Reference
Ataxia telangiectasia	NHL, B-cell, IB [CNS]	11.7%	Gatti [1] Spector [2]
Wiskott-Aldrich syndrome	NHL, B-cell, IB [CNS]	15.4%	Gatti [1] Spector [2]

NHL, non-Hodgkin's lymphoma; *IB*, immunoblastic lymphoma; *CNS*, central nervous system.

Table 2. Iatrogenic cancer

Treatment	Type of tumour	Incidence	Reference
Combined chemo- and radiotherapy	NHL	15%	Krikorian [3]
(Hodgkin's disease)	ANLL	5%	Valagussa [4]
Renal transplant recipients	Skin cancer	4%	Penn [5]
	NHL, B-cell [CNS]	4%	

NHL, non-Hodgkin's lymphoma; *ANLL*, acute non-lymphatic leukaemia; *CNS*, central nervous system.

Table 3. Chronic inflammatory disorders, autoimmune diseases and cancer

Disorder	Type of tumour	Incidence	Reference
Pemphigus	KS and others	12%	Penn [6]
Sjögren's syndrome	NHL	19%	Kassan [7]
Sarcoidosis	(N)HL	11 × normal	Brincker [8]
Endemic malaria	NHL, BL	?	Kafuko [9]

KS, Kaposi's sarcoma; *NHL*, non-Hodgkin's lymphoma; *BL*, Burkitt's lymphoma.

and NHL with B-cell phenotype and central nervous system involvement have been reported.

Chronic inflammatory disorders and so-called autoimmune diseases with complex immunodeficiencies are also associated with an elevated incidence of cancer (Table 3) [6–9]. For example, patients with Sjögren's syndrome have about a 20% risk to develop NHL [7]. There are some reports that the risk of acquiring a malignant lymphoma in sarcoidosis is 11 times higher than in a comparable general population [8]. Kafuko reported a high positive correlation between endemic malaria and NHL especially of Burkitt's type in Africa [9].

To summarize, one can say that there are immunodeficiencies other than those induced by HIV infections which lead to increased incidence of malignant tumours. And it is not astonishing that it is the immune system itself which undergoes malignant transformation. The spectrum of tumour types seems to be similar in most of the described immunodeficiency states. The developing NHL show preferably B-cell phenotypes and have close association with the central nervous system.

HIV Infection and Cancer

Kaposi's sarcoma and malignant lymphomas are by far the most frequently observed tumour types in HIV-infected patients. There is no clear-cut evidence in the literature that the incidence of any other tumours is increased in this type of T-cell deviciency. Nevertheless, there are many reports of single HIV-positive cases in which all kinds of tumours occurred, for example, malignant melanomas, various types of acute non-lymphatic leukaemias and various gastrointestinal carcinomas.

Already in 1982 Lozada observed an increasing incidence of carcinoma of the tongue in young HIV-positive homosexual men in California [10]. There are also two separate reports, one from the United States and one from the United Kingdom, which stress the association of anal carcinoma and homosexuality in HIV-positive individuals [11, 12]. In both types of tumours – oral and anal carcinoma – a viral aetiology is discussed. In the case of anal cancer, as in that of cervical cancer among women, the herpes simplex virus and the human papilloma virus are claimed to play a role in the pathogenesis. It is possible that the T-cell deficiency involved in HIV infection is at least an additional factor in the development of anal cancer.

HIV Infection in Cancer Cases in Switzerland

The preliminary results presented in this paper have been collected by the newly founded Swiss Group for AIDS-Related Tumours, a part of the Swiss Group for Clinical Cancer Research.

To August 1987 a total of 70 patients with Kaposi's sarcoma have been registrated. The simplified map of Switzerland in Fig. 1 presents the geographical distribution of these cases. Forty-six cases have been treated in Zurich, where a total of 644 HIV-positive individuals have been investigated (Rhyner K; personal communication). Those treated in Zurich most probably include some foreigners. This may also be the case in Geneva, a city in which many international organisations are located.

To now 26 cases of HIV-positive malignant lymphomas have been registered in Switzerland: 17 NHL and seven Hodgkin's lymphoma. The geographical distribution of these cases appears somewhat more homogenous than in the case of the Kaposi's sarcoma (Fig. 2).

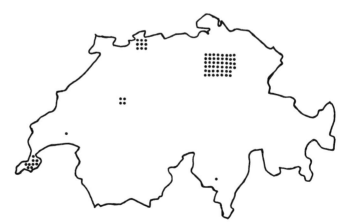

Fig. 1. Geographical distribution of Kaposi's sarcoma in Switzerland (August 1987). Number of cases per canton: *9* Geneva; *1* Vaud; *1* Ticino; *4* Bern; *9* Basel; *46* Zurich; *70* total

Six other tumours were observed in HIV-infected patients to August 1987 (Fig.3). Among these were two patients with testicular carcinomas. As noted above, the relative importance of these few observations remains to be further clarified.

Table 4 summarizes the data collected from Switzerland. In all, 102 malignant tumours of HIV-positive individuals have been registered. These data must be considered very preliminary, since we know that in some regions of Switzerland data collecting has been very incomplete.

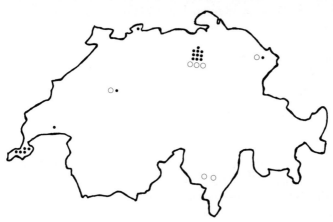

Fig. 2. Geographical distribution of malignant lymphoma in Switzerland (August 1987). Number of cases of non-Hodgkin's lymphoma *(solid circles)* per canton: *5* Geneva; *1* Vaud; *1* Bern; *1* Basel; *10* Zurich; *1* St. Gallen; *19* total. Number of cases of Hodgkin's disease *(open circles)* per canton: *2* Ticino; *1* Bern; *3* Zurich; *1* St. Gallen; *7* total. Sum of malignant lymphomas per canton: *5* Geneva; *1* Vaud; *2* Ticino; *2* Bern; *1* Basel; *13* Zurich; *2* St. Gallen; *26* total

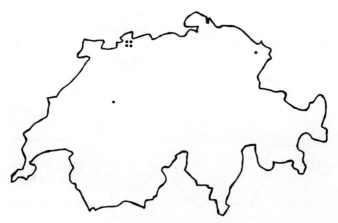

Fig. 3. Geographical distribution of other HIV-related tumours in Switzerland (August 1987). Number of cases per canton: *1* Bern; *4* Basel; *1* St. Gallen; *6* total

Table 4. Cases of HIV infection and cancer in Switzerland by canton in August 1987

Type of tumour	Number of cases per canton							Totals
	GE	VD	TI	BE	BS	ZH	SG	
Kaposi's sarkoma	9	1	1	4	9	46	0	70
Non-Hodgkin's lymphoma	5	1	0	1	1	10	1	19
Hodgkin's disease	0	0	2	1	0	3	1	7
Others	0	0	0	1	4	0	1	6
Totals	14	2	3	7	14	59	3	102

GE, Geneva; *VD*, Vaud; *TI*, Ticino; *BE*, Bern; *BS*, Basel; *ZH*, Zurich; *SG*, St. Gallen.

Table 5. Incidence of non-Hodgkin's lymphoma in Switzerland as of August 1987

Men 1979–1981	8.3 cases/100000 per year
20000 HIV+	Expected: 1.66 per year
	Obseved: 6.33 per year
Ratio Observed/Expected:	3.81
Zurich: 8000 HIV+ Expected:	0.88 per year
	Observed: 3.33 per year
Ratio, Observed/Expected:	3.78

Table 5 shows estimates of the incidence of NHL in HIV-positive individuals in Switzerland. For Swiss men from 1979 to 1981 this was 8.3 per 100000 inhabitants per year (F. Enderlin, personal communication). For the assumed 20000 HIV-positive individuals one would expect 1.66 new tumours per year. In our preliminary analysis we observed 6.33 NHL per year. Thus, the ratio of observed/expected new cases is about 3.8. The same estimation can be made for the region of Zurich (Table 5); the ratio is about the same as for the whole country. Regarding the incidence of Kaposi's sarcoma, no epidemiological data are available for Switzerland.

In conclusion, without any doubt Kaposi's sarcoma and NHL are the most often registered tumours in patients with HIV infection in Switzerland.

References

1. Gatti RA, Good RA (1971) Occurrence of malignancy in immunodeficiency diseases. A literature review. Cancer 28: 89
2. Spector BD, Perry GS, Kersey JH (1978) Genetically determined immunodeficiency disease and malignancy: report from the immunodeficiency cancer registry. Clin Immunol Immunopathol 11: 12
3. Krikorian JG, Burke JS, Rosenberg SA et al. (1979) Occurrence of non-Hodgkin's lymphoma after therapy for Hodgkin's disease. N Engl J Med 300: 452
4. Valagussa P, Santoro A, Kenda R et al. (1980) Second malignancies in Hodgkin's disease: a complication of certain forms of treatment. Br Med J [Clin Res] 1: 216

5. Penn I (1978) Tumors arising in organ transplant recipients. In: Klein G, Weinhous S (eds) Advances in cancer research, vol 28 Academic, New York p 31
6. Penn I (1983) Kaposi's sarcoma in immunosupressed patients. J Clin Lab Immunol 12: 1
7. Kassan SS, Thomas TL, Moutsopoulos MM, et al. (1978) Increased risk of lymphoma in sicca syndrome. Ann Intern Med 89: 888
8. Brincker M, Wilbek E (1974) The incidence of malignant tumors in patients with respiratory sarcoidosis. Br J Cancer 29: 247
9. Kafuko GW, Burkitt DP (1970) Burkitt's lymphoma and malaria. Int J Cancer 6: 1
10. Lozada F, Silverman S, Conant M (1982) New outbreak of oral tumors, malignancies and infectious diseases strikes young male homosexuals. Calif Dent J 10: 39
11. Daling JR, Weiss NS, Klopfenstein LL et al (1982) Correlates of homosexual behavior and the incidence of anal cancer. JAMA 247: 1988
12. Peters RK, Mack TM (1983) Patterns of anal carcinoma by gender and marital status in Los Angeles Country. Br J Cancer 48: 629

Inactivation of HIV and Safety Precautions for the Workplace*

B. R. Saltzman and A. E. Friedman-Kien

Kaplan Cancer Center, Department of Medicine, New York University Medical Center, 550 First Avenue, New York, NY 10016, USA

In June 1981 the initial reports of the occurrences of *Pneumocystis carinii* pneumonia and Kaposi's sarcoma in previously healthy homosexual men [1, 2] heralded the beginning of the epidemic now known as the acquired immune deficiency syndrome (AIDS). Shortly thereafter it was recognized that the particular populations found to be at risk for the development of AIDS – homosexual or bisexual men, intravenous drug users, hemophiliacs, and people who have received blood transfusions or other blood products – were also known to be at risk for infection with hepatitis B (HBV).

Previously designed safety precautions to limit the transmission of HBV in health care settings were used as a model for the development of infection control guidelines for dealing with patients with AIDS, even before the true infectious nature was known and the etiologic agent of the syndrome, the human immunodeficiency virus (HIV) was identified [3, 4]. The isolation of HIV and the subsequent development of specific and reliable serologic tests for detecting antibodies to the virus provided the means for studying the epidemiology of the disease and the modes of HIV transmission.

The three main routes of transmission of HIV are: (a) sexual contact, (b) blood-borne via transfusion with infected blood or blood products (e.g., factor VIII clotting concentrates) or sharing of blood-contaminated needles in the practice of intravenous drug use, and (c) perinatal transmission from an HIV-infected mother to her newborn child. HIV has been isolated from blood, semen, vaginal and cervical secretions, saliva, tears, breast milk, cerebrospinal fluid, amnionic fluid, and urine, and it is likely to be found in other body secretions and excretions [5]. Each of these body fluids is potentially infectious, although the specific routes of entry and the actual concentration of viral particles in the inoculum may play significant roles in determining the efficiency of transmission of HIV due to contact with these fluids. Epidemiologic evidence suggests that direct parenteral exposure to infected blood and sexual contact with exchange of semen, vaginal secretions, or blood appear to pose the greatest risks of contracting HIV infection [6, 7].

Close, nonsexual contact such as that which occurs in the household setting is associated with minimal to no risk of HIV transmission. None of the more than

---

* This manuskript was supported by the Howard Gilman Foundation and the Samuel and May Rudin Foundation, both of New York.

50000 cases of AIDS reported to the Centers for Disease Control (CDC) by February 1988 has occurred in family members of patients with AIDS, unless the members have had other recongnized risk-related behavior. Traditionally nearly 500 family members of patients with AIDS were evaluated in seven published studies. Family members frequently engaged in extensive sharing of household items and facilities, and close personal interactions over prolonged periods of time. In spite of this, these studies failed to demonstrate a single HIV infection among household members who did not have additional exposure to HIV through blood, sexual activity, or perinatal transmission [8].

As the prevalence of HIV infection and AIDS throughout the world continues to increase, there is a greater chance of individuals coming into contact with HIV-infected persons, including asymptomatic carriers. On the other hand, contact with saliva appears to be associated with a low risk of HIV transmission [8].

In Vitro Inactivation of HIV

The virus HIV itself is highly labile and has been shown to be readily inactivated in vitro. HIV may be inactivated by heat, desiccation, alkalinization or acidification, and by exposure to a variety of germicides or disinfectants (Table 1). The virus may be heat-inactivated at 56 °C in aqueous solution. the precise time required for complete inactivation of the virus at 56 °C has been reported to range from 10 min to 3 h [9-11]. The differences in these observations may be due to variations in the concentration of the serum or viral particles in the preparations tested, or they may perhaps be related to the type of in vitro assays employed in each of the studies. Total inactivation of HIV maintained in a dried state at ambient room temperature (24°-26 °C) required from 3 to 7 days; however, a 2 log decrease in the tissue culture 50% infectious dose ($TCID_{50}$) of the dried virus was reported to occur within 6 h at room temperature [11]. The virus has also been shown to be inactivated by exposure to acid or alkaline conditions, but was found to be somewhat more readily inactivated in vitro at low pH than at high pH [9].

HIV has been shown to be rapidly inactivated by exposure to commonly used germicides or disinfectants at concentrations much lower than those generally employed [9, 13] (Table 2). The agents which have been tested and shown to be effective in inactivating HIV include: a 0.1% dilution of household bleach; 50% ethyl alcohol; 35% isopropyl alcohol (rubbing alcohol); 1% glutaraldehyde (Cidex); 0.5% paraformaldehyde; 0.5% Lysol (active ingredients: soap, 16.5%; *o*-phenyl phenol, 2.8%; *o*-benzyl-*p*-chlorophenol, 2.7%; alcohol, 1.8%; xenol, 1.5%; isopropyl alcohol, 0.9%; and ethylenediaminetetraacetate, 0.76%); 1% neutral buffered formalin; 0.25% povidone iodine (Betadine); and 1% solution of the nonionic de-

Table 1. Inactivation of HIV

1. Heat – 56 °C for at least 10 min
2. Drying at room temperature
3. pH
4. Germicides and disinfectants

Table 2. Inactivation of HIV: germicides and disinfectants

Agent	Effective concentration (%)	Commonly used concentration (%)
Household bleach	0.1	10
Ethyl alcohol	50	95
Isopropyl alcohol	35	70
Glutaraldehyde	1	2
Paraformaldehyde	0.5	1
Lysol	0.5	3
Neutral buffered formalin	1	10
Povidone iodine	0.25	10
Nonidet P-40	1	0.5

tergent Nonidet P-40 [9–13]. The durations of exposure required for complete inactivation of HIV by each of the various disinfectants range from less than 60 s up to 10 min. Other agents shown to inactivate HIV include nonoxynol-9, an agent commonly used in contraceptive spermicides; sodium oxychlorosene (Clorpactin), an antibacterial agent; and tri(n-butyl) phosphate/sodium cholate, a combination of an organic solvent and a detergent [14–16]. Standard methods for sterilization and disinfection employed in laboratories and health care settings are more than adequate to inactivate HIV.

Health Care Workers and Allied Professionals

Health care workers are potentially at higher occupational risk for HIV infection than the general work force, as they are more likely to be exposed to HIV-infected blood and body secretions and with greater frequency in the performance of their jobs.

Health care workers and allied professionals, including students and trainees, whose occupational activities may involve contact with blood and other body fluids, include but are not limited to: physicians, nurses, hospital aides, dentists, dental hygienists and assistants, optometrists, podiatrists, chiropractors, clinical and research laboratory staffs, especially blood bank technicians, phlebotomists, dialysis personnel, paramedics, emergency medical technicians, forensic pathologists and their assistants, hospital housekeepers, and laundry workers [17].

Studies of occupationally acquired HIV infection show the risk to be quite small. Prospective evaluation of 1594 health care workers following parenteral or mucous membrane exposure to potentially infected blood or body fluids of HIV-infected patients in four large population based studies documented only four individuals infected with HIV who had no other risk factors for infection (0.3%) [5, 18–21]. A seroprevalence study of dentists and dental workers found one dentist out of a population of 1309 (0.08%) who had antibodies to HIV in the absence of other risk factors [22]. Of note was the fact that this dentist was often exposed to blood and saliva, rarely used gloves in his work, and suffered multiple needlesticks in the course of his practice, but never knowingly treated an HIV-infected patient. There have also been anecdotal reports of nine other health care providers who have evidence of occupationally acquired infection with HIV. Three of these individuals were health care workers with percutaneous needlestick exposure to HIV infected blood or body fluids [23–25], one was a health care worker with mucous membrane exposure, and two were health care workers with nonparenteral exposure [25], two were care providers with prolonged extensive but nonparenteral exposure to infected materials [27–28]. The ninth individual was a technician in a research laboratory who was exposed to HIV in a much higher concentration than that encountered in a clinical setting [28].

While the patterns of transmission of HIV are similar to those of HBV, the efficiency of transmission of HBV is much greater. The risk of acquisition of infection from a single needlestick from an HBV infected patient ranges from 6% to 30%, as compared to a less than 1% risk of HIV infection associated with a single needlestick contaminated with blood from an HIV-infected patient [17].

The latency period for developing clinical disease following infection with HIV may be as long as 7 years or more [30]. It is therefore difficult, if not impossible, to identify all asymptomatic, seropositive individuals with whom a health care worker may come into contact. It is essential that individuals involved in health care consider all patients as potentially infectious for HIV and observe recommended infection control measures when handling all blood or body fluids.

Recommended Infection Control Guidelines

Protective Attire. Health care workers should wear appropriate protective attire when coming into contact with blood or body fluids from all patients, not only from those believed to be infected with HIV. Disposable gloves should be worn whenever drawing blood or coming into contact with body fluids, mucous membranes, or tissue specimens. Disposable or sterilizable gowns should be worn in circumstances in which accidental splashes of blood or body fluids may occur; masks and goggles should be worn when performing procedures in which spray or aerosolization of body fluids might happen.

Hand washing between contacts with patients and after handling blood or body fluids should be a strict rule, even after the removal of disposable gloves. Health care workers with open skin wounds, cuts, or denuded excoriated, eczematous, or exudative dermatitis, especially involving their hands, should refrain from direct patient care or handling of patient blood, body fluids, or contaminated medical instruments and other equipment until their skin disorder has totally healed.

Disposable Needles and Surgical Blades. Whenever possible, disposable needles, syringes, surgical blades and other instruments should be used. Extreme care should be taken in the disposal of needles, syringes, and surgical blades, since the greatest risk for HIV infection to health care workers has been shown to be due to percutaneous exposures, 40% of which were potentially preventable [18]. Used needles should *not* be recapped, bent or clipped; rather they should be discarded directly into conveniently located puncture-resistant trash containers that are specially and clearly labeled as containing biohazardous or infectious material to alert unsuspecting employees who may handle such containers. These disposable containers should be constructed so that the contents, once inserted, cannot be removed or fall out. As a further precaution, the containers should be autoclaved prior to disposal or incinerated [5].

Immediately following any accidental spilling of blood or body fluids, contaminated surfaces should be immediately wiped up and cleaned with a proper disinfectant.

Potentially High-Risk Health Care Situations

Specific infection control guidelines for several health care settings require special mention: the dental office, dialysis units, autopsy rooms, morgues and mortuaries, and clinical and research laboratories.

Dental Office. Dental workers should wear gloves for all contact with oral mucous membranes of all patients. In addition, they should wear surgical masks and protective eyewear or chin-length plastic face shields for any procedures in which splashing or spattering of blood or saliva frequently occurs. Rubber or plastic disposable dams, a shieldlike drape often used by dentists during oral surgery, should be utilized when appropriate to minimize the generation of droplets and spatter. The removable handpieces of dental instruments such as drills should be autoclaved or sterilized with appropriate disinfectant after use with each patient. Ideally, the dentist's office should be equipped with several such handpieces, so that some 'may be undergoing sterilization as the others are in use. Handpieces that cannot be sterilized should be flushed and the outside surface cleaned with a suitable disinfectant after use. All nondisposable surgical instruments, including bone chisels, picks, scalers, and scissors should be heat-sterilized after each use [5, 31].

Dialysis. Patients infected with HIV who require dialysis may undergo either hemodialysis or peritoneal dialysis, whichever is clinically indicated. There is no need for these patients to be isolated from other patients. The standard infection-control practices currently employed in dialysis units are sufficient to prevent the spread of HIV infection [32].

Autopsy Rooms, Morgues, and Mortuaries. All persons performing or assisting in postmortem procedures including autopsies and embalming should wear gloves, masks, protective eyewear, disposable gowns, and waterproof aprons and footwear, which can be cleaned with a disinfectant. Instruments and work surfaces contaminated with patient tissues and body fluids or excrement during postmortem examinations should be rigorously cleaned with an appropriate chemical germicide [5]. Tissue biopsy specimens that are fixed in formalin, which inactivates HIV, can be handled in the usual manner without danger of infection [12]. However, frozen histologic sections of tissue which are not fixed in formalin must be treated with infection-control precautions. The microtome blades used in slicing the fresh frozen tissues must be sterilized after use.

Clinical and Research Laboratories. In the laboratory, all persons processing blood and body fluid specimens should wear disposable gloves. In addition, face masks, goggles, and gowns should be worn when working with patient tissue blood or body fluids in situations in which spatter or splashes may occur, or when performing HIV isolation procedures, including tissue culture. Biological safety laminar flow hoods or cabinets should be used whenever procedures are conducted that might have a high potential for generating HIV-infected droplets in the laboratory. These laboratory procedures involve activities such as centrifuging, blending, sonicating, and vigorous mixing. Tissue culture and HIV propagation should also be done in biological safety cabinets. Production of large quantities or high concentrations of HIV must be performed only in special laboratories with appropriate isolation precautions (biosafety level 3) [33]. In the laboratory, oral pipetting must never be employed, for fear of accidental ingestion of infected fluids. Mechanical automatic suction pipetting apparatuses with disposable pipettes must routinely be employed for diluting, aliquoting, or transferring any blood, serum, or other potentially infected fluids to disposable test tubes or other laboratory wares. All residual tissue and body fluid specimens and the contaminated containers should be either autoclaved or incinerated before final disposal in a health department approved sanitary manner.

Office or Hospital Invasive and Diagnostic Procedures. Gloves should be worn by physicians and surgeons as well as by any other medical professionals performing invasive diagnostic patient procedures, such as endoscopy colonoscopy, bronchoscopy, cystoscopy or skin, bone marrow, or liver biopsies. Gowns, masks, and goggles should be worn if there is a possibility of excessive bleeding or spraying with blood or body fluids [34]. Instruments used in these procedures should be either disposable or adequately sterilized prior to reuse on another patient. Surgeons and operating room assistants should wear a second pair of latex gloves as an extra precaution against accidental cuts or tears during surgery.

Other Occupations at Potential Risk for Exposure to HIV Infection

Employees of correctional facilities, custodial institutions, nursery schools, and child day-care centers may be unknowingly exposed to asymptomatic HIV-infected individuals. The employees who come into close contact with potentially infected persons should take appropriate glove and gown infection-control precautions when involved in situations in which there is exposure to blood, body fluids, or excretions.

Personal Services Providers. Individuals who provide services in nonhealth care settings which might put them into contact with blood or body fluids should also observe guidelines to limit the possible transmission of HIV. This recommendation applies to barbers, hairdressers, manicurists, cosmeticians, masseurs, and people performing electrolysis, tatooing, acupuncture, and ear piercing [17]. To date, there has been no documented transmission of HIV to or from a personal service worker or through client-to-client contact in the course of providing such services.

All reusable instruments, including razors, scissors, cuticle and nail clippers, and needles or piercing equipment should be adequately disinfected following each use, either by autoclaving or placing in an appropriate germicide for at least 10 min. Ideally, single-use disposable instruments such as razors and acupuncture and piercing needles should be used. Personal service workers may require more than one set of instruments so that one may be undergoing disinfection while the other is in use. Blood from any accidental nicks or cuts should be promptly wiped up and cleaned with a readily available disinfectant (alcohol or bleach). Personal service workers should use disposable latex gloves to protect themselves from accidental injury and potential infection as well.

Potential Transmission of HIV from Health Care Workers to Patient

There has been no documented transmission of HIV from an infected health care provider to a patient. This route of infection is theoretically possible, especially if the infected health care worker sustains a cut or puncture wound in the course of performing an invasive procedure, thereby contaminating the open wound of the patient. The issues of widespread testing of health care workers for HIV infection and how to act on a positive result remain controversial. It has been suggested that an HIV-infected health care worker should elect to refrain from performing invasive procedures [5, 17].

Universal Precautions

With the exception of the child born to an HIV-infected mother, individuals currently uninfected with HIV have it within their power to remain uninfected. In the case of health care workers and personal service workers, this requires concerted efforts to decrease contact with body fluids by observing appropriate precautions. To achieve this goal, educational programs to teach about HIV infection, modes of transmission, and necessary infection control procedures must be implemented in the in-service settings and in professional schools. Such educational efforts may also help to diminish exaggerated and irrational fears regarding HIV infection and improve overall patient care services. Although costly, protective attire must be used when coming into contact with any body fluid from *all* patients. Gloves must be worn for all blood drawing, dental examinations, minor surgical or invasive procedures, and when handling any laboratory specimens. Each patient and every specimen must be considered potentially infectious. Health care workers must not be lulled into a false sense of security by only treating known or suspected HIV-infected individuals with the appropriate precautions [5].

References

1. Gottlieb MS, Schroff R, Schanker HM et al. (1981) *Pneumocystis carinii* pneumonia and mucosal candidiasis in previously healthy homosexual men: evidence of a new acquired cellular immunodeficiency. N Engl J Med 305: 1425
2. Friedman-Kien AE, Laubenstein L, Marmor M et al. (1981) Kaposi's sarcoma and *Pneumocystis pneumonia* among homosexual men – New York and California. MMWR 30: 250–252
3. Barre-Sinoussi F, Chermann JC, Rey F et al. (1983) Isolation of a T-lymphotropic retrovirus from a patient at risk for acquired immune deficiency syndrome (AIDS). Science 220: 868–871
4. Popovic M, Sarngadharan MG, Read E, Gallo RC (1984) Detection, isolation and continuous production of cytopathic retroviruses (HTLV-III) from patients with AIDS and pre-AIDS. Science 224: 497–500
5. Centers for Disease Control (1987) Recommendations for prevention of HIV transmission in health-care settings. MMWR 35 [Suppl 2S]: 3–18
6. Ward JW, Deppe DA, Samson S et al. (1987) Risk of human immunodeficiency virus infection from blood donors who later developed the acquired immunodeficiency syndrome. Ann Intern Med 106: 61–62
7. Curran JW, Morgan MM, Hardy AM et al. (1985) The epidemiology of AIDS: current status and future prospects. Science 229: 1352–1357
8. Friedland CH, Klein RS (1987) Transmission of the human immunodeficiency virus. N Engl J Med 317: 1125–1135
9. Martin LS, McDougal JS, Loskoski SL (1985) Disinfection and inactivation of the human T lymphotropic virus type III/lymphadenopathy-associated virus. J Infect Dis 152: 400–403
10. Spire B, Barre-Sinoussi F, Montagnier L, Chermann JC (1984) Inactivation of lymphadenopathy associated virus by chemical disinfectants. Lancet: 899–901
11. Resnick L, Veren K, Salahuddin SZ, Tondreau S, Markham PD (1986) Stability and inactivation of HTLV-III/LAV under clinical and laboratory environments. JAMA 255: 1887–1891
12. Martin LS, Loskoski SL, McDougal JS (1987) Inactivation of human T-lymphotropic virus type III/lymphadenopathy-associated virus by formaldehyde-based reagents. Appl Environ Microbiol 53: 708–709
13. Kaplan JC, Crawford DC, Durno AG, Schooley RT (1987) Inactivation of human immunodeficiency virus by betadine. Infect Control 8: 412–414
14. Hicks DR, Martin LS, Gretchell JP et al. (1985) Inactivation of HTLV-III/LAV-infected cultures of normal human lymphocytes by nonoxynol-9 in vitro. Lancet ii: 1422
15. Klein RJ, Buimovici-Klein E, Ong KR, Czelusniak SM, Lange M, Friedman-Kien AE (1987) Inactivation of human immunodeficiency, herpes simplex, and vaccinia viruses by sodium oxychlorosene. Lancet ii: 281–282
16. Prince AM, Horowitz B, Brotman B (1986) Sterilisation of hepatitis and HTLV-III viruses by exposure to Tri(n-BUTYL)phosphate and sodium cholate. Lancet 706–710
17. Centers for Disease Control (1985) Recommendations for preventing transmission of infection with human T-lymphotropic virus type III/lymphadenopathy-associated virus in the workplace. MMWR 34: 681–686, 691–695
18. McCray E (1986) The Cooperative needlestick surveillance group. Occupational risk of the acquired immunedeficiency syndrome among health-care workers. N Engl J Med 314: 1127–1132
19. Henderson DK, Saah AJ, Zak BJ, Kaslow RA, Lane C et al. (1986) Risk of nosocomial infection with human T-cell lymphotropic virus type III/lymphadenopathy-associated virus in a large cohort of intensively exposed health care workers. Ann Intern Med 104: 644–647

20. Gerberding JL, Bryant-LeBlanc CE, Nelson K, Moss AR, Osmond D et al. (1987) Risk of transmitting the human immunodeficiency virus, cytomegalovirus, and hepatitis B virus to health care workers exposed to patients with AIDS and AIDS-related conditions. J Infect Dis 156: 1–8
21. McEvoy M, Porter K, Mortimer P, Simmons N, Shanson D (1987) Prospective study of clinical, laboratory, and ancillary staff with accidental exposures to blood or other body fluids from patients infected with HIV. Br Med J [Clin Res] 294: 1595–1597
22. Klein RS, Phelan A, Freeman K et al. (1987) Low occupational risk of human immunodeficiency virus infection among dental professionals. N Engl J Med 318: 86–90
23. Anonymous (1984) Needlestick transmission of HTLV-III from a patient infected in Africa. Lancet: 1376–1377
24. Oksenhendler E, Harzic M, Le Roux JM, Rabian C, Clauvel JP (1986) HIV infection with seroconversion after a superficial needlestick injury to the finger. N Engl J Med 515: 582
25. Neisson-Vernant C, Arfi S, Mathez D, Leibowitch J, Monplaisir N (1986) Needlestick HIV seroconversion in a nurse. Lancet 2: 814
26. Centers for Disease Control (1987) Update: human immunodeficiency virus infections in health care workers exposed to blood of infected patients. MMWR 36: 285–289
27. Centers for Disease Control (1986) Apparent transmission of human T-lymphotropic virus type III/lymphadenopathy-associated virus from a child to a mother providing health care. MMWR 35: 76–79
28. Grint P, McEvoy M (1985) Two associated cases of the acquired immune deficiency syndrome (AIDS). PHLS Commun Dis Rep 42: 4
29. Weiss SH, Goedert JJ, Gartner S et al. (1988) Risk of human immunodeficiency virus (HIV-1) infection among laboratory workers. Science 239: 68–71
30. Hessol NA, Rutherford GW, O'Malley PM et al. (1987) The natural history of human immunodeficiency virus infection in a cohort of homosexual and bisexual men (Abstract). In: Abstracts from the III international conference on AIDS, June 1–5, 1987, Washington, DC, p 1
31. Centers for Disease Control (1986) Recommended infection-control practices for dentistry. MMWR 35: 237–242
32. Centers for disease control (1986) Recommendations for providing dialysis treatment to patients infected with Human T-lymphotropic virus type III/lymphadenopathy-associated virus. MMWR 35: 376–383
33. Centers for disease control (1986) Human T-lymphotropic virus type III/lymphadenopathy-associated virus: agent summary statement. MMWR 35: 540–549
34. Centers for disease control (1986) Recommendations for preventing transmission of infection with human T-lymphotropic virus type III/lymphadenopathy-associated virus during invasive procedures. MMWR 35: 221–223

Psychosocial Issues for Patients with AIDS-Related Cancers

H. Christ

Department of Social Work, Memorial Sloan-Kettering Cancer Center,
New York, NY 10021, USA

The social and psychological aspects of acquired immunodeficiency syndrome (AIDS) are almost as complex and challenging as the biological. Its onset affects every aspect of a patient's life; it may cause serious problems for those with whom the patient has personal, intimate familial, or occupational ties; it produces difficult patient management issues for health care institutions and community agencies; and it raises basic ethical issues for the health care community as long as the contagious potential of the disease remains. The complexity of problems confronting people with AIDS and the terror it invokes set this disease apart from virtually every other contemporary public health problem.

Last year a young lawyer in a large corporation office was diagnosed with AIDS on the basis of visible Kaposi's sarcoma lesions on his neck and hands. Although he was well-liked and respected, his situation created considerable tension among the office staff, who viewed his presence as a threat to their well-being. In spite of legal support, reassurance by experts that his disease could not be causally transmitted, and al although he was a valuable employee who still felt physically well, he was finally compelled to leave work when his secretaries refused to touch his papers.

The most recent study of the age of AIDS patients shows that 53.6% are in the 34–54 age range, and that 39% are between 15 and 34 years of age [1]. They engage in a broad range of occupations, a fact that often challenges stereotypes held about where they work. Therefore, the developmental issues confronted by persons with AIDS are those of a young, socially and emotionally vulnerable population, often in the most productive years of their lives: not unlike the psychosocial issues confronting individuals diagnosed with leukemia.

The patient's progress in fulfilling the developmental tasks of young adulthood is profoundly challenged by the demands of AIDS and its treatment. These tasks include choosing an occupation, establishing a career, forming enduring intimate relationships, solidifying ones sense of identity, and establishing and refining an adult life pattern. A very familiar and often successful coping strategy is for the patient to make a supreme effort to continue his/her development in these areas until physical limitations absolutely prevent continuation. Work is often viewed by the young adult patient as a statement of value, identity, self-worth, and an assurance of some "normalcy." And, in addition, it protects private medical insurance. Therefore, many patients try desperately to conceal the signs of their disease in order to be able to work as long as possible.

Recent Results in Cancer Research, Vol. 112
© Springer-Verlag Berlin·Heidelberg 1988

The Need for Primary Prevention

A major emphasis on primary prevention has developed in the United States over the past year as the numbers of patients have continued to increase, the prevalance levels in identified risk groups have become high, and there are indications of spread into the much larger heterosexual population. Research on prevention in the Department of Social Work at Memorial Sloan-Kettering Cancer Center has demonstrated how very difficult it is for young, highly educated individuals engaged in high-risk behaviors to accept the degree of their vulnerability and to make effective changes until in many cases, it is too late. In our research in the Department of Social Work we found that 5 years into the epidemic 48% of the asymptomatic gay men in our sample were continuing high-risk practices [2].

Preventive-education efforts have reached some of these individuals, but many have made changes that are insufficient to protect them, given the current prevalence of AIDS among homosexual men. Handsfield has pointed out that the prevalence is cumulative. Therefore, for example, in San Francisco where it is estimated that perhaps two-thirds of the homosexual population are HIV-positive, an individual reducing his sexual contacts from ten to two per year, using only unprotected sex, will still have an 89% chance of exposure to the virus [3]. We have also observed that in the face of such an enormous threat individuals use a broad range of cognitive distortions of facts and idiosyncratic health schemas that lead them to underestimate their risk and in some instances to adopt behavior changes that are not efficacious, for example, while many individuals continue to follow safer sex guidelines following a negative HIV test, others reason that since they were exposed but have not yet contracted the disese they must have an immunity to it, and they may therefore continue or increase high-risk behaviors.

Until an effective cure or immunization against AIDS is developed, the principal strategy for controlling its spread will be through persuading at-risk, infected, and diseased populations to modify behaviors implicated in the development and transmission of the disease. While the majority of AIDS patients are still homosexual or bisexual men, the number of patients contracting the disease through intravenous drug use and heterosexual contact, especially women, is increasing. As a result of these recent changes in transmission routes, we have found it essential to encourage a focus on high-risk behaviors rather than on high-risk groups. Viewing infected individuals as belonging to certain high-risk groups, i.e., homosexual men or intravenous drug users, rather than as individuals who practice high-risk behaviors has enabled many to deny their vulnerability if they do not belong to these groups. It allows one to feel safe if not a member of such groups, rather than encouraging a realistic assessment of risk-taking behaviors. It is what one does, not what group one belongs to that determines one's risk. Therefore, AIDS is an issue for all sexually active individuals who are not in long-standing, mutually monogamous relationships.

Psychosocial Impact of AIDS on Patients and Their Sexual Partners

From a psychosocial perspective, individuals affected by AIDS can be viewed as being at different points along a health-illness continuum: those worried but well, those at risk, those known to be HIV-positive, and those symptomatic with either ARC or AIDS. Each of these points along the health-illness continuum confronts the individual with specific social and psychological challenges that he or she must adress. This paper focuses primarily on those social and psychological issues that confront both the patient, especially the patient who has AIDS and cancer, and the sexual partner of the patient.

Issues Confronting the Patient

Disclosure of Life-style/Diagnosis to Family, Friends, and Employers. While individuals who are HIV-positive are able to confine this information to those who must know about it, e. g., sexual partners, once they are diagnosed AIDS patients, they need to tell more people about their disease. This is necessary in order to obtain financial benefits, to deal with work and social absences due to medical treatment and illness, and to explain physical changes. Patients worry about whom to tell, who suspects, and who in knowing their secret will reject them, and they need to discuss this decision-making concerning disclosure with staff. However, talking with health professionals about their illness can also lead to discussing sexual and drug behaviors that they may have hidden. This is a particularly difficult struggle, for example, for bisexual men. Philip, a 40-year-old successful businessman, had kept his bisexuality a secret from his wife, child, parents, and business associates. When he became ill and needed people to help him, he worried about whom the could tell, and about what they would think of him.

Need for Confidentiality. Persons with AIDS may be quite reluctant to share personal information because of fear of loss of confidentiality leading to the loss of jobs and insurance and because of overt social discrimination. They may be extremely hesitant to give information until they feel secure that their confidentiality will be maintained, and that they are respected and accepted by the professional. Physicians and other health professionals can help patients by directing them to identify those individuals in their personal network whom they most trust and by helping them develop effective ways of communicating. These experiences of social discrimination are often very real, and patients may need to ventilate their fear and anger about such occurrences. Finally, the physician and other health professionals can also help by advocating for the patient when they do experience discrimination, actively interceding on their behalf with employers or with friends and family.

Loss of Self-Esteem. When the individual becomes an AIDS patient, real physical differences occur, such as extreme weight loss, visible Kaposi's sarcoma lesions, loss of energy, and other body changes. Patients struggle with tremendous loss of self-esteem over these changes. Those who have Kaposi's sarcoma lesins live with a constant visual reminder of the disease which interferes with adaptive denial. The lesions also heighten the feeling of stigma and evoke physical distance to and rejection by others. Finally, the appearance of many lesions can signify to the patient the failure of the immune system and disease progression. For example, patients describe being terrified when they are taken off anticancer chemotherapy because of immune suppression, and suddenly the lesions reappear all over their body. At that point, they may demand to be started on chemotherapy again even if their body is exhausted and vulnerable to infection from it. For these reasons patients are often more preoccupied with the cosmetic treatment of their lesions than with efforts to treat the underlying disease. They may request radiation therapy of their lesions before they begin chemotherapy.

The loss of work and the social isolation caused by such visible and aversive signs of disease are profoundly disturbing to patients. They try to cover the lesions with makeup, which can be very effective; however, as the lesions progress, this may become less effective and make them look even more conspicious. Patients are faced with needing to mourn their lost attractiveness and physical and social desirability and may be helped by being allowed to be open about such grief. Lee, a 28-year-old architect, said, "I can't look at myself in the mirror. I don't know whose face that is. I look ugly and dead already."

Anxiety About an Uncertain Disease Course. The uncertainties in the disease course are also stressful to patients, leading to their feeling like a "walking time bomb," just waiting for the next medical crisis or "explosion" to occur. They wonder whether they should continue working or go on disability benefits in the face of such uncertainty, even if at the moment they are feeling well. However, they fear that leaving work will confront them with a lack of purpose and meaning in their lives. Therefore, patients frequently push themselves to continue even though it may be physically quite difficult, until the day when they, in fact, cannot physically go into work and realize that they cannot return. This is a common coping strategy for the young adult. A major therapeutic goal is to help patients cope with this uncertainty through directing them to concentrate on those aspects of their experience that are within their control. They can be encouraged to use intellectual defenses, such as closely monitoring the course of the disease, developing means of relaxation and anxiety control, and ventilating their fears and concerns.

Fear of Abandonment and Isolation. Patients' fears of abandonment are exacerbated when family, friends, and colleagues are frightened by the nature of the disease, by different life-styles, and by the confrontation with death and therefore distance themselves over long periods of time. If friends are also at risk for getting the disease, the identification with a patient may cause them to withdraw from contact with him. Patients can be helped by learning to open up communication with those friends and relatives who are able to continue involvement with the patient. They can also be helped by referral to a range of community agencies that have been developed for the express purpose of providing social networks and helping individuals who are isolated because of their disease. In New York the Gay Men's Health Crisis Center is such an agency that was developed by the homosexual community, and in San Francisco the Shanti organization provides a large number of individuals, usually volunteers, who are able to be personally and socially available to patients. Although, the intravenous drug user community is not as well organized, and services for these patients are more limited, self-help groups and drug treatment centers also provide for them.

Fears of Separation, Loss, and Death. Fears associated with a potentially fatal illness are common to AIDS patients. They fear the loss of life time, their peers "getting ahead" of them, and their being unable to "catch up." Patients are depressed about the loss of potential in what they could have done and might have become; they are depressed about the loss of their dreams.

Patients may rarely talk of their feelings about being ill and concentrate instead on the issues of keeping their job, maintaining their home, and family and friend relationships. They may emphasize any aspect of their condition which would help them avoid acknowledging that they have AIDS. For example, they cling tenaciously to the fact that they have swollen glands, pneumonia, tuberculosis, or cancer. The patient who has lymphoma, a cancer less frequently associated with AIDS, and is also HIV-positive will frequently talk only about his or her cancer. In this situation, cancer is seen as less stigmatizing and more hopeful than AIDS. This defense of adaptive denial should be respected until the professional can assess the individual's coping pattern. Bill, a 40-year-old postal clerk, was so convinced that he had cancer, and not AIDS, that he confused physicians who met him for the first time. Upon exploration, it was learned that his lover had died of AIDS, an experience so horrifying to him that he could not accept his own diagnosis.

Denial can be a useful and necessary defense for patients with a fatal illness because it gives them a control over when and how they will confront their own mortality. For AIDS patients, however, denial is less likely to be effective because of the extensive media coverage of the disease. It is hard for patients to turn on a television or radio or read a newspaper without hearing that AIDS is incurable. In addition, patients are also often demoralized by the death of other AIDS patients they have known.

Even at the terminal stage of illness some patients may choose not to discuss their thoughts and fears about death with professional staff. In fact, most patients state that they are more afraid of the process of dying – the pain, the discomfort, the symptoms of central nervous system disease, and disfigurement – than of death itself. Health professionals therefore need to be open to such discussions, but not feel compelled to push the patient to discuss these issues, especially during the earlier illness stages.

Recurring Suicidal Thoughts. Thoughts of suicide are common among AIDS patients and are usually related to their anger, their fear of being isolated, and their concerns about being unable to manage the symptoms and the progress of their disease. Patients often state that, ... if "I will kill myself if I get much sicker," ... if "I am unable to work," ... if "I am in pain," or "... if the AIDS goes to my brain." Fears of the symptoms of an incurable illness can provoke intense feelings of helplessness and hopelessness. While the professional is always apprehensive about suicide, it seldom occurs with AIDS patients if they are allowed to ventilate their feelings, are assured that they are cared for, and can clearly see that they will have options at every phase of the illness – even terminal illness – e. g., pain medications will be made available to them, and they will have choices about their treatment and choices about life-sustaining procedures. Their sense of control in the disease and the treatment experience needs to be maintained. In addition, it is very important to ensure that patients have adequate social contacts with individuals in the community to limit their degree of isolation and aloneness, which can provoke suicidal thoughts.

Greg, a 36-year-old clothes designer, presented as depressed and having suicidal thoughts. When given the opportunity to talk about his feelings, Greg confided that his worst fears were not having medical insurance or money to pay for his rent and buy food. When he was helped to obtain some financial assistance, his feelings of vulnerability and helplessness were diminished.

It is necessary, of course, to obtain a history of prior suicidal thoughts from individuals who have AIDS and to assess their previous coping patterns and behavior in this area. Patients are often very reassured by the active involvement and concern from medical staff.

Central Nervous System Disease. Increasing numbers of patients have been found to have symptoms of central nervous system disease, characterized by a progressive dementia that can become severely incapacitating [4]. Early symptoms may include memory loss (names, historical details, appointments), difficulty with concentration (losing track of conversation or in reading), mental slowing (less quick, verbal spontaneous), and confusion of time and of persons [5]. The patient may also appear apathetic, withdrawn and "depressed." A minority of patients demonstrate a more agitated state, with hyperactivity and inappropriate behavior. Unsteady gait, leg weakness, loss of coordination, impaired handwriting, and tremor are also possible early manifestations.

As the symptoms progress, patients may need extensive help with the activities of daily living. These include traveling to and from the hospital, preparing meals, and many aspects of personal care. Patients fear these symptoms, which they view as "going crazy" or being "demented" almost more than any other. Loss of memory and mood changes elicit deep sadness and intense anger. Therefore, patients may attempt to conceal such symptoms when possible by not communicating them to their physician and by removing themselves from situations in which they might be exposed. Instead, they may discuss them with another member of the health care team or with a caretaker.

Tim, a 35-year-old musician, yelled at his friends and then refused to talk to them on the phone and discouraged them from visiting him. When the social worker discussed this with him, he said, "I just don't have the patience to figure out their questions, and I just don't remember what the doctor says to me."

Useful interventions for management of these symptoms related to the central nervous system include the following.

1. In discussing this disease with a patient, physicians should present the symptoms of central nervous system disease as a possible aspect of the patient's experience, emphasizing those particular symptoms that respond to treatment. We

strongly recommend that health professionals avoid terminology that has become particularly frightening, such as "dementia."

2. Close communication with the patient's caretaker and other health team members may enable early identification of such symptoms. It may be quite helpful for the physician to determine with the patient, soon after diagnosis, who the responsible caretaker of the patient is. Knowing this early facilitates making plans for the patient's care, should he or she experience cognitive impairment. Both physician and caretaker must do this sensitively, with an understanding of ways of working with the patient's adaptive denial.

3. Once these symptoms have emerged, it may be necessary to provide an ongoing assessment of the adequacy of the supervision in the patient's home environment in the present of these cognitive and physical changes.

These cognitive changes also have a tremendous impact on patients' relationships with people close to them and with professional staff. Early in the course of the AIDS epidemic central nervous system disease symptoms were not diagnosed in their milder form. Rather, they were interpreted by both professionals and individuals close to the patient as psychological reactions to being diagnosed with the disease [5]. Because of this, caretakers often found the patient's withdrawal, depression, and anger, which they believed to be controllable by the patient, as behavior impossible to tolerate. Many of the caretakers felt the development of these behaviors to be a "last straw." In other words, the patient was blamed for poor coping. Early identification of central nervous system disease symptoms facilitates timely supportive treatment when possible, for example, psychotropic medications for depression, anxiety, and other psychiatric symptoms. It also allows for the provision of adequate care for the patient in his home and enables both professional staff and the patient's caretakers and friends to be more effective in their care and support of the patient.

Later symptoms of AIDS dementia can include psychomotor slowing to virtually absolute mutism [6]. The ataxia and clumsiness of gait may give way to paraparesis, and urinary and fecal incontinence can occur. The patient may be confined to hed in the end stage, staring vacantly about and capable of only the most rudimentary social or intellectual interaction [6]. These symptoms often necessitate the patient's institutionalization during the terminal illness because home care becomes too complex for most families or caretakers to manage.

Lymphoma and Other Cancers. Lymphoma and other cancers diagnosed in patients who are also HIV-positive is a relatively new medical condition [7]. While these patients must acknowledge their HIV infection and their potential for infecting others, they frequently demonstrate significant denial of their AIDS-related condition, preferring to identify themselves as cancer patients; an example is that of Bill, described above ("Fears of Separation, Loss, and Death"). Such defensive denial should be respected until the professional can assess the person's coping patterns and strengths.

It may be difficult to obtain needed financial assistance for patients if they are unable to acknowledge their AIDS-related condition and apply for AIDS-specific benefits. Intervention strategies with such patients often need to accept the patient's denial to a certain extent and at the same time assist the patient in realistic planning for his present and future care. Patients who demonstrate strong denial early in the illness may experience increasing distress as the symptoms of AIDS become more apparent during terminal illness, as the patient's denial is no longer effective, and he/she confronts the AIDS diagnosis for the first time.

Psychosocial Issues for Partners of AIDS patients

Decision-Making Concerning Sexual Relationships. The sexual partner of a person with AIDS is confronted with the specter of losing someone he or she loves and depends on. At the same time, such partners are confronted with fears about their own exposure to the virus and the possible risk to their children. Beth, a 32-year-old real-estate agent, upon learning that her boyfriend was diagnosed with AIDS began to scream that she too wanted to be ill so that they could "die together." Several weeks later when she agreed to be tested for exposure to the virus, she said she hoped God had not heard her first request!

Developing safer sexual practices is a tremendous challenge to the relationship when there is such fear. Initially these practices seem artificial, nonspontaneous, and "too clinical." Couples often need help in discussing ways to remain physically close. As patients become more debilitated, their sexual needs and abilities are, in fact, diminished. Partners react with sadness and anxiety, as the change in sexual relationship is symbolic of the impending greater loss. It is not unusual for these young patients to fear losing their partner because they can no longer satisfy him/her sexually. Without open discussion of these issues they may begin to erode the couple's relationship, making them feel isolated, angry, and increasingly fearful of the future.

The need to change sexual patterns is a special problem for women, especially women in minority groups, among whom the disease is rapidly rising in the United States. They have little sense of sexual entitlement, i.e., a sense of a right to direct the sexual relationship. Refusing sex often means losing income, housing, child care, and often the only source of human contact.

Guilt About Possibly Having Transmitted the Disease. All sexually transmitted diseases have the component of guilt or blame on the part of the individual who brought the disease into the relationship, especially when one partner is sexually active or is using drugs outside the relationship and even if they both knew about this behavior. For instance, Cathy, a 35-year-old bookkeeper, said she knew that Angelo had used drugs before they met, and that she could accept this, but she never bargained for his getting AIDS. She related her feeling both love and hate for him.

Concern About Partners' Health and Worry About Ones Own. In addition to learning about safer sexual practices, it is helpful for partners to maintain and to monitor their own health as a way of gaining a sense of control at such a difficult time. They need to be able to discuss symptoms in confidence with a physician in order to contain their anxiety.

Issues Relating to Communication, Warmth, Closeness, and Intimacy. All couples must deal with maintaining communication and intimacy in the face of serious illness and fears of loss and separation, whether the relationship is traditional or nontraditional. Gerri and Stuart met at a homosexual club. Neither had ever experienced a long-term relationship. As they both became ill, their relationship became closer, less focused on sex, and more focused on tenderness and mutual concern. Counseling helped them realize the depth of their concern for each other.

Decisions About Childbearing. Finally, decisions about childbearing are influenced by facts and by religious, cultural, and personal values. This is one of the most troubling issues for individuals who are HIV-positive. Many women who are HIV-positive choose to have a child, risking their own and their child's life, as they view this as their only source of fulfillment in life. Others choose to have an abortion or decide to remain childless, a profound psychological challenge for both men and women.

Summary and Conclusion

The social, psychological, and ethical challenge of AIDS, specifically AIDS-related cancers, is as complex as the biological and medical. Both the patient and his or her sexual partner experience a number of stresses to which they must adapt. AIDS also poses a challenge to professionals and to the social fabric of countries in which it occurs.

One test of the worth of a society is the way in which it handles its fears, its sick, and its stigmatized individuals. The challenge to us all is to respond to this disease, to those endangered by it, to those overwhelmed by their fear, and to those who contract it with the clarity of thought, scientific excellence, high ethical standards, and human compassion that enables all of us to continue life with dignity and meaning.

References

1. AIDS surveillance update. New York City Department of Health AIDS Surveillance Unit, preliminary data.
2. Siegel K, Christ GH, Moynihan RM, Krown S, Gold J, Safai BJ, Sordillo P (1987) Patterns and correlates of change in sexual behavior among homosexual men at risk for AIDS. Paper presented at the annual meetings of the American Society of Clinical Oncologists, Atlanta, Georgia
3. Handsfield HH (1987) AIDS and sexual behavior in gay men. Am J Public Health 17: 329–350
4. Nemia BA, Jorden BD, Price RW (1986) The AIDS dementia complex: clinical features. Ann Neurol 19 (6): 517–524
5. Beresford TP, Blame FC, Hall RCW (1986) AIDS encephalitis mimicking alcohol dementia and depression. Biol Psychiatry 21: 394–397
6. Rosenblum M, Sidtis J, Price RW (1987) The AIDS dementia complex: some current questions. Ann Neurol: (in press)
7. Lowenthal DA, Straus DJ, Campbell SW, Gold JWM, Clarkson BD, Koziner B (1987) AIDS-Related lymphoid neoplasia: the Memorial Hospital experience. Cancer (manuscript submitted)

Summary and Future Prospects

L. Schmid

Abteilung für Onkologie und Hämatologie, Medizinische Klinik C,
Kantonsspital St. Gallen, 9007 St. Gallen, Switzerland

The data on the association between infection with the human immunodeficiency virus (HIV) and malignant tumours presented in Stein an Rhein can be summarized briefly as follows:

1. The incidence of HIV infection is increasing rapidly in the United States of America and in Central Europe. Data on the increase in the number of malignant tumours in HIV infected individuals are incomplete.
2. Kaposi's sarcoma is part of the acquired immunodeficiency syndrome (AIDS), and the variant in AIDS patients is more aggressive than the classical one. Nevertheless, progression of Kaposi's sarcoma is only rarely limiting in the course of AIDS. If treatment is indicated, radiotherapy is in many cases effective.
3. Non-Hodgkin lymphoma is also closely associated with HIV infection. Typical features of these lymphomas are the highly malignant morphology with a B-cell phenotype, the high rate of extranodal localisation (CNS) and the high proportion of advanced stages (III and IV). It is possible that the incidence of other tumour types such as Hodgkin's lymphoma is also increased in HIV-infected patients.
4. An acceptable rate of complete remission of highly malignant non-Hodgkin lymphoma in HIV-positive individuals can be achieved with aggressive combined chemotherapy. Unfortunately, the data presented by various authors show very short median survival times (5–6 months). Patients die from opportunistic infections as well as from progression of the tumour.

In the near future our knowledge of HIV-induced immunodefects may also have some effect on the understanding of the pathogenesis of virus-associated malignant tumours.

Since there are no good treatment modalities for HIV infection, prevention of further transmission of the virus is the only method that will be successful in the fight against this disease.

For patients with highly malignant tumours such as non-Hodgkin lymphoma alternative therapeutic strategies should be elaborated and tested in prospective cooperative trials. Combinations of conventional cytostatic regimens with drugs which can at least temporarily reverse the HIV-associated immunodefects would be one of the possibilities in this field.

Subject Index

abandonment, fear 87
acidification 76
acquired immunodeficiency syndrome
  (AIDS) 20f.
  associated conditions 39
  in Central Europe 1ff.
  CMV infection 59
  development 17
  epidemic 6, 11, 27, 56, 75
  etiology 6ff.
  HIV-seropositive subjects 46
  Hodgkin's disease 38, 40f.
  immunological mechanisms 17
  life expectancy 29
  malignant lymphomas 37ff.
  neoplastic complications 37
  non-Hodgkin's lymphomas 13, 38ff.
  pathogenesis 8, 17
  patients, family members 75f.
    psychosocial issues 84
    sexual partners 86, 91f.
  related complex (ARC) 20f., 39f.
    complications 18
    neoplasias 6
    tumors 71, 84
      Swiss Group 71
  risk groups 28
  statistics 1
    current infection rate 4
adriamycin 34
α-interferon 34
alkalinization 76
alkylating agents 54
angiolipoma 11
antibody, neutralizing 20
antigenic stimulation, chronic 17
ataxia telangiectasia 6, 54, 69
autoantibodies to T-cells 18
autoimmune responses by HIV-proteins 10
autopsy rooms 79

azathioprine 54
azidothymidine (AZT) 35

behaviour, high-risk 85
biopsies, lymph node 58
bleomycin 34
blood transfusion 27, 47, 75
B symptoms 57f.

cancer 90
  incidence 11
  oral 11
  rectal 11
  skin 7
carcinoma
  anal 12, 37, 71
  anorectal 71
  cloacogenic 56
  gastrointestinal 71
  genital 12
  hepatocellular 12
  of the lung 11
  of the mouth 56
  nasopharyngeal 12, 56
  testicular 11, 56, 72
  of the tongue 37, 56, 71
cells
  antigen presenting (APC) 8
  HIV-infected 9
  killer 8
    natural (NK) 18, 21
  supressor, activity 18, 21
chemotherapy 34, 69
  aggressive combined 58, 93
  combined with antiretroviral drugs 59
  infectious complications 34
  and NHL 55
childbearing 92
coagulation intravascular disease 41f.
colony stimulating factors (CSF) 59

communication 92
cooperative trials, prospective 93
coping strategy 87
corticosteroids 54
cryotherapy 34
cyclosporin A 54
cytomegalovirus (CMV) 12, 17
cytotoxicity, antibody dependent cell-mediated (ADCC) 10, 18, 21

damage, central nervous system, HIV-associated 10
death-fears 88
defect, immunological 17
denial, adaptive 88, 90f.
dental office 79
desiccation 76
diagnostic procedures 80
dialysis 79
diethyldithiocarbamate (DTC) 22
dinitrocholorbenzene (DNCB) 34
disclosure of diagnosis 86
disease
    autoimmune 54f., 70
    central nervous system 88
    immunodeficiency 54
    inflammatory 54f.
disinfectants 76f.
drug abusers 47

Epstein-Barr virus (EBV) 12, 17
etoposid (VP16) 34

fear of abandonment 87
    death 88
    isolation 87
    loss 88
    separation 88
France 46
future prospects 3, 93

genes, regulatory 7
germicides 76f.
γ-interferon 8
guilt 91

health care workers 77f.
health care situations, high-risk 79
heat-inactivation 76
hemophiliacs 27, 75
herpes simplex virus (HSV) 17
heterosexual contact 47
    population 2
histocompatibility complex, major (MHC) 9

Hodgkin's disease 11, 47, 63, 70f.
    AIDS-related 58
    extranodal manifestations 43
    mixed cellularity-type 65
    in patients with HIV-infection 57
homosexuality 47
homosexuals 2, 38
    AIDS-associated Kaposi's sarcoma 28
    chronic active infections 17
    CMV-infection 12
    HIV-positive 71
    Kaposi's sarcoma 27, 75
    malignant lymphoma 38
    pneumocystis carinii pneumonia 27, 75
HTLV-IV, pathogenic potential 7
human immunodeficiency virus (HIV)
    antiviral immune responses 10
    classification 6
    genome 7f.
    inactivation 75ff.
    infected cells 9
    infection
        B-cell hyperplasia 13
        immunological characteristics 17
        immunotherapy 17
        and malignant lymphoma 54ff., 63ff.
        occupationally acquired 78
        risk for exposure 80
        and tumors 11
    proteins 7f.
    seropositive subjects 21, 46, 90
        childbearing 92
        and Kaposi's sarcoma 12
    transmission 75, 85
        from health care workers to patient 81
hypergammaglobulinemia 18f.

immune
    activation 17
    antiviral responses 10
    chronic stimulation 54
immunity, defective, cell-mediated 27
immunodeficiency 54, 69
    congenital 55
    T-cell 21, 69
immunomodulation therapy 22
immunorestorative therapy 22
immunosuppression, chemical 54
infections
    activation of latent DNA-virus 12
    chronic active 17
    control 78
    HIV, incidence 93
    opportunistic 7, 18, 27, 37, 40ff.

infections
    treatment 35
inflammatory disorders, chronic 70
intravenous drug addicts 2, 27, 38, 75
    chronic active infections 17
    Kaposi's sarcoma 3
    malignant lymphomas 38
interleukin 2, 8
isolation, fear 87
Italy 37

Kaposi's sarcoma 6, 11 f., 18, 20, 37, 55, 69,
    71, 93
    AIDS-related 27 ff.
        risk groups 28 f.
        treatment 34
    CMV-associated 12
    differential diagnosis 33
    endemic 12
    epidemic 28
    etiology 33
    HIV-related 12
    in intravenous drug abusers 3
    and malignant lymphoma 56
    in organ transplant recipients 12
    sporadically ocurring 12

laboratories 80
LAV-2, pathogenic potential 7
leukemia
    acute 69
        non-lymphatic 69 ff.
    prolymphocytic 56
lymphadenopathy
    angioimmunoblastic 40
    HIV-associated 58
    lymph node biopsies 58
    persistent generalized (PGL) 38 ff., 58
lymphocyte, T-, cytotoxic (CTL) 18, 21
lymphokine 8
lymphoma
    AIDS-related 56
        management 58
    malignant 63, 71, 90
        anorectal 59
        Burkitt-type 12, 37, 42, 57, 65
        centroblastic 65
        centrocytic 65
        EBV-induced 18, 57
        and HIV-infection 54 ff., 57 f., 63 ff.
        immunoblastic 6, 37, 65
        and Kaposi's sarcoma 56
        lymphoblastic 37, 65
    in patients with AIDS 38

non Hodgkin's (NHL) 6, 11, 13, 37, 47,
    55, 69 ff., 93
    B-Cell 6, 13, 18, 70
    CNS-origin 37 f., 42, 56
        differential diagnosis 59
    extranodal location 37, 39, 43, 56
    high-grade 54
    incidence 72
    initial site 39 f.
    primary, of the brain 11
    thymic 12

malignancy
    AIDS-related 55 f.
    hematological 46
    high-grade 63
    intermediate-grade 63
    low 63
melanoma, malignant 71
morgues 79
mortuaries 79
multiple myeloma 56

neoplasia
    hematological 46
    HIV-related 46

oncoviruses, human 11
organ involvement 64, 66

papilloma virus, human 12
persistent generalized lymphadenopathy
    38 ff.
plasmocytoma 64 f.
    solitary 56
pneumonia, pneumocystis carinii 27
population, sexually promiscuous 11
potential risk, persons exposed to 5
precautions 75 ff.
    universal 81
prevention 93
    primary 84
professionals, allied to health care 77 f.
psychosocial impact 86

radiotherapy 69
recommendations to persons exposed to po-
    tential risk 5

safety 75 ff.
self esteem 86
separation, fears 88
serum immunoglobulins 66
sexual partners 86, 91

suicidal thoughts 88
summary 93
survival, median 93
Switzerland 69, 71
syndrome, Wiskott-Aldrich 6, 69

T-cell
  depletion 18, 57
  helper 8
  immunodeficiency 57
  perturbed function 18
therapeutic strategies, alternative 93
therapy
  antiretroviral 35, 59
  immunomodulatory 22ff., 35
  immunorestorative 22ff., 60
  immunosuppressive 6, 27, 54f.
  non toxic 24
T-lymphocytic, cytotoxic (CTL) 8
transplant recipients

and Kaposi's sarcoma 12
  organ 55
  renal 6, 27, 69
treatment 64, 67
  cosmetic 87
trends, certain population groups 2
tumors
  DNA-virus associated 12
  in HIV-infections 11
  "secondary" 69
  skin 69

uncertainty in disease course 87

vinblastine 34
viral effects
  indirect 10
  on HIV infected cells 9

workers, health care 77f.